Triumphs of the Human Spirit

Triumphs of the Human Spirit

Real Cancer Survivors,
Real Battles,
Real Victories

Barry W. Summers

Writers Club Press
San Jose New York Lincoln Shanghai

Triumphs of the Human Spirit
Real Cancer Survivors, Real Battles, Real Victories

Writers Club Press
an imprint of iUniverse, Inc.

For information address:
iUniverse, Inc.
5220 S. 16th St., Suite 200
Lincoln, NE 68512
www.iuniverse.com

Disclaimer: The author is not a medical doctor, and does not have any formal medical training. The author believes that all information in this book is true, complete and accurate. However, he makes no warranty or guarantee to that effect. Neither the author nor the publisher shall be liable for any claim, damages or other result, including but not limited to illness or death, which may result from following any of the procedures described in this book.

ISBN: 0-595-20904-1

Printed in the United States of America

To Lorri and Rachael
For Everything

CONTENTS

SELMA SCHIMMEL FOREWARD

You are about to read stories of survival and inspiration. These are human stories illustrating the power of transformation. I am one of these stories, and together our hope is that wherever you are in your healing, you discover the possibility of something maybe even better than before.

It is certainly not that one wants to get cancer to achieve something meaningful or extraordinary with his or her life, it's just that when any one of us is seriously challenged, another way to work with it is to make it work for you. That is what you'll find here. And to varying degrees and in different ways it exists in every one of us.

I am very fortunate to be able to talk to so many people about their attitudes and feelings about cancer. I remember the first time a discussion about the difference between being healed and being cured took place on *The Group Room*® radio show. I was deeply moved because of its profound and simple truth, and that being cured of cancer is not the same thing as being healed of cancer.

As you read these personal life essays of survival, the common theme of integrating the cancer experience into one's life is fundamentally clear. When you live in fear and when you lock your feelings inside of yourself, it is yet another toxic malignancy within. Any one of us who embraces our survival or decides to become a cancer advocate on any level is reinforcing the self-claimed benefits and rewards that we create *with* and *because* of cancer in our lives.

When Barry Summers asked me to write the foreword for his book, it was a great honor for me. The most important message he wants to get across, especially to the newly diagnosed, is the back-to-life strength shown by survivors who are excelling, and that you not only can survive cancer, but that you can thrive as well.

When cancer throws you the curve ball, what are you going to do? If you grab it with determination, one step at a time, know that a diagnosis of cancer does not define who you are and that you are not alone; survival takes on a whole new meaning.

It is what you do with the cancer that matters so much more than what the cancer does to you. It is surely different for everyone and there will be losses to bear. You might not get what you want, but you can create something else. But, there is work involved; whether you have cancer or someone you love and care about does, you have to also have the courage to talk about it and not isolate yourself.

Use resources, reach out for support, and remember that dreams and hope are ever changing constants in our lives.

Selma Schimmel—

Founder and President, Vital Options

ACKNOWLEDGEMENTS

First, I'd like to thank the two greatest inspirations I've ever seen:

Terry Fox, 1958-1981, who died while on a run across his native Canada on an artificial leg. He died 16 years before I was diagnosed, but I've never forgotten how he showed the world that a cancer survivor could be tougher than anyone, cancer or not. Second, Lance Armstrong, world-class cyclist and three-time Tour-de-France winner. He beat metastatic testicular cancer with a 3% chance of making it. He put himself into the 3% group. I am so honored to have his story in my book. Someone said of Lance, "He is hope."

I'd also like to thank the many other cancer survivors who are beating it every day. I wish I could put everyone in my book. I'd like to thank my father Jordan Summers, who beat bladder cancer without giving it another thought, and to acknowledge my father-in-law, Dave Werbo, who beat Non-Hodgkin's Lymphoma and still makes jokes about it.

I also want to acknowledge the fact that yes, people do die of cancer. I wish I could have met Terry Fox, and I'd like to thank Dr. Harry Klein, who I'd known for 20 years. He went through kidney cancer before I did, supported me and was happy to live to see me get my black belt. He died two months later and his wisdom will never leave me. I'd also like to thank "BACE", who went through kidney cancer and was the survivor who helped get me through the process. Another loss mourned is my kidney, whom I've named "Righty Summers," and a death in any form is real if you're going through it.

Huge thanks go out to my friends and colleagues at Ortho Biotech, who were extremely supportive of my efforts to write this book. And what's more, big thanks for making my job a pleasure to go to every day. Nothing beats low stress to help extend your life. Thanks to Bob Roach, Carol Goodrich, and especially Carol Webb for believing in the value of this project. Also, my gratitude to Linda Seekamp for her great transcriptions and ideas; Kassy McGourty who did so much; Megan Brocail for her beautiful editing; Peter Murphy who captured on film exactly what I wanted my cover picture to say; and Bob and Terri Albrecht who put up with me throughout the design process. Also to the professionals at iUniverse.com who moved things along so quickly, and to the many charities and organizations named in this book who cooperated so much. Also to Congressman Jim Greenwood for his help, time and consideration. And, of course, to the hundreds of people I interviewed for this book. Of the nearly fifty stories that appear on these pages, my favorite is "all of them."

I'd like also to thank my friends, my wife Lorri, my daughter Rachael, my family, and to my honored teachers in Philly and Temple University who helped make me the person I am today. My greatest teachers, though, were my karate senseis, too modest to want their names in print—I'll just say Walt, who taught me about power; Phil, who taught me to breath; and Ron, who taught me everything else.

Many thanks, also, to those who make every day a little easier: Howard Stern for my laughs driving to work, Opie & Anthony for my laughs on the drive home, and to the Three Stooges and John Fogerty who kept my mind off recovering from surgery.

My eternal gratitude to the people who do the research to create the diagnostic equipment, drugs and treatments for all diseases, America is the greatest country in the world for medicine because of you. I want to thank the world-class medical team I had: Dr. Lewis Dunn and Dr. Adelina Dunn for the flawless care and for yelling at me for not moving fast enough, and as always, Sue and the ladies in the office who took care of everything; Dr. Ron Summers, MD, PhD, for my second opinion and the best brother a guy could have and of course Nancy E.F. Summers for all her cancer research and for being a great friend and sister-in-law

On a separate line, I have to thank Hector I. Ramirez, a powerful spirit and an unforgettable presence to anyone who has ever met him.

To the nurses, staff, interns, residents, fellows, lots of other doctors, and everybody else who run the show at Thomas Jefferson University Hospital in Philadelphia, I couldn't change a thing if you paid me. Last but never the least, Dr. Stephen Edward Strup, Thomas Jefferson Urology Associates, for his excellent medicine, surgery, bedside manner and mementos. If it had been my time to go, the Lord would have sent me somewhere else.

The two last people I want to thank are the most important: My daughter Rachael who came along just two years ago, who makes every day better than the last and continues to remind me what's so great about this life. I saved the best for last, Lorri Summers, RN BSN for being the best girlfriend, wife AND nurse—you are the funniest person I've ever known and the 'best date' a guy could ever ask for. Thanks for putting up with me, for believing in the book, for pushing me on, and for making my life complete. Also, for making sure I take my vitamins and for making me eat a salad every day. I told you when we met that our life would be an adventure, didn't I?

Charity from the sale of this book goes to the Kimmel Cancer Center Advocacy and Survivorship Program for patient support at Thomas Jefferson University. For more information they can reached at 215.955.8370 or on the web at *www.kcc.tju.edu*. An equal amount also will benefit the Urinary Tract Cancer Research fund (kidney, bladder, prostate, testis, etc) of the Thomas Jefferson Urology Associates.

For information on discounts for group/charity bulk purchases of this book, please email Bulk Whole/Sales at bws1@mindspring.com.

COVER PHOTO: Peter Murphy.
Cover Photo shows the author standing in the Delaware River outside of Lambertville, New Jersey, in front of his newest hobby, his rowing club.

INTRODUCTION

Triumphs of the Human Spirit
   Real Cancer Survivors, Real Battles, Real Victories

Find the good. It is all around you. Find it, showcase it, and you'll start believing in it—Jesse Owens

Welcome to The Club.

No, it's not an organization into which you're inducted based on your social status, superior intellect nor athletic prowess. And, when you're called to join, it's not an invitation you can readily refuse.

The "club" I'm referring to is cancer survivors, a society of more than 9 million Americans brought together by a single diagnosis. Bound together by the fight they have been through. And we are a very unified group. We're not interested in differentiating between ourselves, and we are very colorblind. If only the rest of the world felt this way!

The common thread in the Club members' stories I've captured in this book isn't their hazing—the surgery, chemotherapy, hair loss and radiation treatments. It's not their religious beliefs, their support networks nor their souls. Their common bond is their invincible spirit.

Having survived cancer, I know that there is a distinct difference between your soul and spirit. Your soul is what you get for free. Your spirit is what you do with it.

If you are diagnosed with cancer and survive, you've won a great fight. But the triumph comes with what you do with your victory. And, as my own surgeon articulated, "You'll be a cancer survivor until the day you die from something else."

Right now, if you've been newly diagnosed, you know about people who have died or people who have 'made it'. Maybe you are hearing more negative news than you are positive. When I was diagnosed, everyone tried to think of how many people they knew who died from it. Oh boy, what encouragement. I am here to tell you that 9 million people are surviving, and many of them are doing even better.

If you can learn anything from this book, it's that you *can* survive cancer. But you can go to the next level, too: you can *thrive* beyond cancer. And while no one, myself included, would ever voluntarily seek membership into The Club, I can guarantee that surviving cancer will be the most transforming experience of your life. It *can* be a great transformation. If I could contribute one thing to the world as it fights cancer, it would be to change everyone's perception: you don't have to be afraid of cancer. It isn't necessarily a death sentence.

As you read this book, you may not relate to everyone's experiences or their philosophical approaches. But if just one passage helps you to believe that you, too, can be victorious over cancer, not just survive, then I will have fulfilled my purpose.

If, at this point in your diagnosis, you are not ready to read further, let me at least provide you with the 10 previously unwritten bylaws of The Club, as professed independently by just about every contributor to this book.

1. Cancer isn't necessarily a death sentence.

2. You're not alone. You're an ordinary person in an extraordinary situation.

3. Don't ask, "Why?" Ask, "What now?"

4. Medical statistics are for doctors, not survivors.

5. Your doctor's not the final judge.

6. Knowledge is stronger than fear.

7. Cancer isn't as fatal as a loss of hope.

8. Cancer doesn't build character; it reveals it.

9. If you wake up breathing, it's a good day.

10. Sometimes, you just have to laugh.

I'm going to add one more: Ask, Argue and Advocate—be a partner with your doctor, make your own decisions where you can, and don't passively accept something you don't like. Get the best doctor you can and fight like hell.

For those of you who choose to read further, keep your heart and mind open. If you hear a statistic, believe that you will be on the winning side. Then help somebody who's been diagnosed even more recently than you have, and tell them the same thing: triumph over cancer is not only a desirable goal, but a very attainable one as well. Don't just aim for survivorship; aim for what I'd call 'thrivorship'.

Barry Summers
Author and Cancer Survivor
March 29, 2001

Triumphs of the Human Spirit

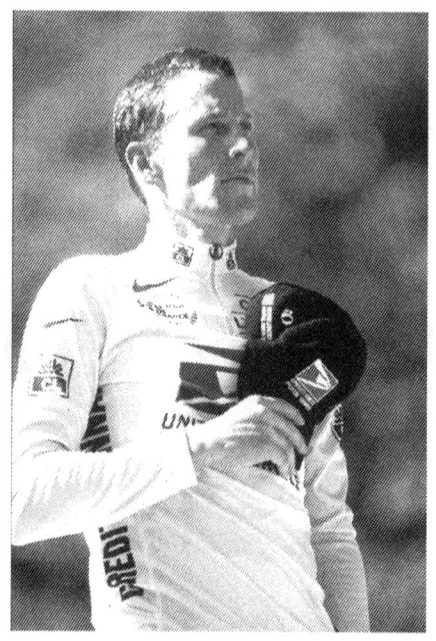

Lance Armstrong, 29

Married 2 years to Kristin, son Luke (1).

World-class cyclist, winner of the 1999, 2000 and 2001 Tour de France, a 2100 mile bike race over the mountainous perimeter of France. Author of the autobiography "It's Not About the Bike."

Born: Austin, TX; Live: Austin, TX.

Tumor Type: Testicular, with metastases to the brain and lungs, diagnosed October 2, 1996.

Treatment: Surgery to remove testicle and brain lesions, plus Chemotherapy.

The Lance Armstrong Foundation (on the web at laf.org) raises money for cancer research.

Photo Credit: Graham Watson, showing Lance receiving final award of the 1999 Tour De France, as the American Flag is raised and the national anthem played.

HEART OF A CHAMPION

Many parallels can be drawn between the ups and downs and rigorous nature of cancer survival and the famous Tour de France bicycle race.

Cycling 2100 miles through mountainous terrain, treacherous weather and against the greatest cyclists in the world could be considered somewhat of a death-defying feat. But it's nothing compared to fighting cancer.

In his book, *It's Not About the Bike*, testicular cancer survivor Lance Armstrong said he was positively challenged by the odds against him; in short, he likes a good fight. Cancer made a big mistake when it picked him, and he fought the cancer mentally as well as physically, every day.

For example, to cope with the pain and discomfort of chemotherapy, he visualized his coughing and his burning urine as tumors being scorched and leaving his body.

Lance credits his recovery to his unyielding belief. He was told after his recovery that his doctor had secretly thought he had only a three percent chance of surviving. Even if his doctor had shared his fear, Lance would not have given up. He believes that anything is possible, as long as you pledge to fight the battle. In his case, Lance fought by educating himself about the disease, constantly seeking out new information, along with second and third opinions, and learning about every possible cure that might be available to him.

He does caution, however, that even after effective physical treatment, a person's soul needs time to heal. In dealing with the emotional effects of cancer, the feeling of being alone hits home and hits hard. Lance reminds us that with 8 million Americans living with some form of cancer to reach out to, no one should feel isolated.

Lance's victory in the Tour de France had a profound effect on people around the world, whether cancer survivors or not. Lance's victory was the greatest symbol that you don't just survive cancer, you can thrive. Sure, we all have our doubts and the fear of recurrence is always hovering in the back of our minds. But for Lance and all other survivors, the celebrated expression, "The greatest revenge is living well," should guide us not only on the journey to recovery, but on the much more rewarding journey ahead.

Whether the fight is won or not, Lance believes that we are always much better than we think we are. Our true capabilities emerge in time of crisis, and the process itself makes us a better and stronger person.

And if you, like Lance, can also believe that cancer improves us, it shouldn't be considered a form of death, but a part of life.

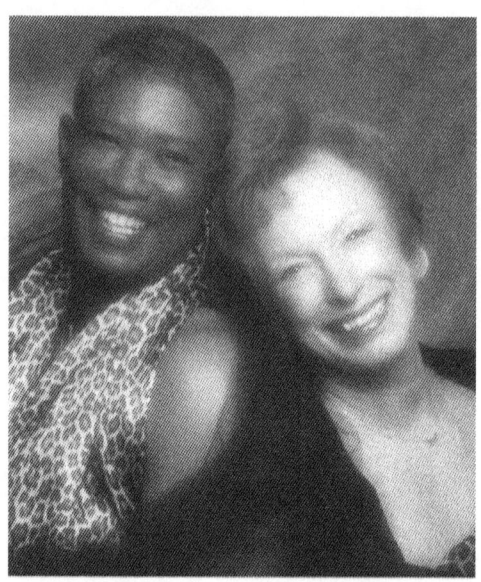

Sandra Jackson, 51 and Mimi Williams, 62

Sandra has been dating Paul Brown for 9 years; Mimi has been dating Vito Lentini for 4 years. Mimi has four children and Sandra has two.

Sandra and Mimi run 'Courage Unlimited', a non-profit organization in Las Vegas "that's not just for cancer survivors but for anyone with a health challenge."

Sandra Born: New York, NY. Live: Las Vegas, NV

Mimi Born: Chicago, IL. Live: Las Vegas, NV

Tumor Type: Breast cancer in 1992 (Mimi) and 1993 (Sandra). Sandra had metastases to the lungs and a breast cancer recurrence in 1995.

Treatment: Lumpectomy and partial mastectomy with radiation (Mimi). Radical modified mastectomy, chemo and radiation for breast cancer and lobectomy for lung cancer (Sandra).

You can learn more about the ladies and their show at www.courageunlimited.com.

Photo Credit: Kelley Sweet for the "Wall of Hope."

WHAT COLOR IS YOUR CANCER?

"I came from a privileged background and didn't realize that cancer can strike anybody—it doesn't discriminate based on your age, sex or economic status," explains Mimi Williams. "After my diagnosis, I stopped caring about what people were wearing and driving, and tried to see their heart."

Mimi and her best friend and cohort, Sandra Jackson, are both breast cancer survivors, who now host "Courage Unlimited," a television talk show in Las Vegas. They also sponsor the "Essence of Beauty" survivors' magazine and yearly retreat.

"I just couldn't believe it happened to me," Mimi recounts. "I was healthy, exercised, delivered and nursed my four kids before the age of 30—nothing ever indicated that I might be a candidate for breast cancer."

Mimi was a model for most of her life, so the idea of losing a breast was devastating. "Before my diagnosis, I never considered that there was a lot more to me than just my body."

Her friend and cohost concurred. "Between my mastectomy and subsequent hysterectomy, I thought, 'Who would want me?'" Sandra recalls. She then experienced a recurrence, this time in her lung. "I was terrified of the lung cancer because cancer was not in my family at all." Her third recurrence was in her chest wall, requiring surgery.

Mimi and Sandra discuss bonding with all fellow cancer survivors. "When I'm hurting, I can call Mimi or I can call anyone who has had breast cancer to say, 'I just need to talk to you.' and the person on the other side can say, 'I understand where you're coming from,'" Sandra expressed.

Her experience has also taught her that cancer doesn't discriminate. "A lot of people try to play this color thing. When I woke up from my first surgery I had two white women standing over me. I don't know if there were any African-American women available to speak to me at that time, nor did I care. What I wanted was a sister to hold my hand and let me cry," Sandra remembers. "When we began our television show, we got race out of the way by asking each other 'what color is your cancer?'"

Cancer has transported Mimi to the core of her spirituality. "It's a wonderful trip just opening up more and more of the healing that can happen through recognizing how important your spirituality is. The little messages you get in the most innocent ways are like a guiding spirit," Mimi said.

She added, "Healing is about energy. You cannot have negative energy around you if you are in a healing process because you will not heal mentally or physically. Give out positive energy. What others do with it is their choice."

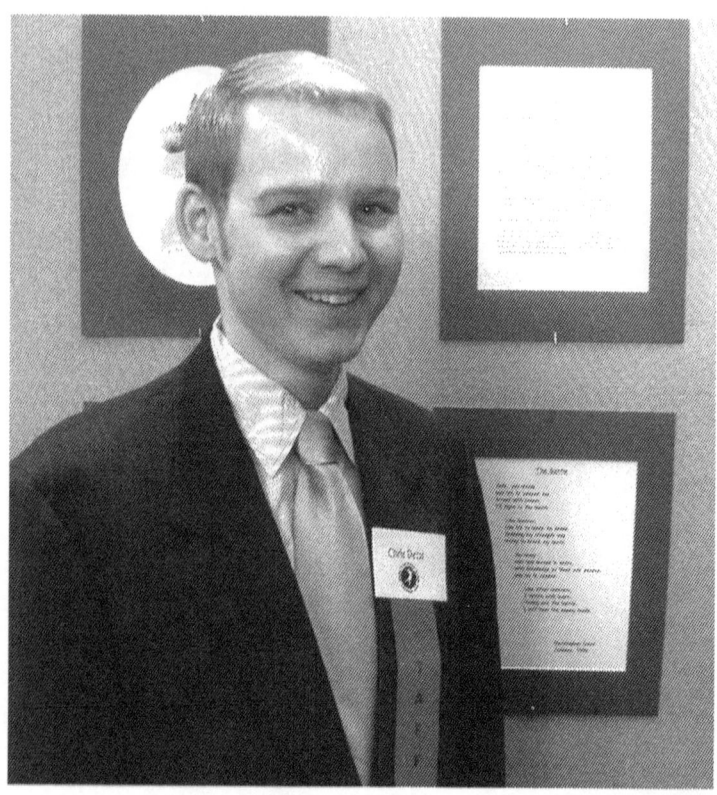

A. Christopher Dezzi, 27

Engaged to Kathy Wood, RN.
Chris is Vice President of the Dezzi Group, political and business consultants.
Born: Philadelphia, PA. Live: Philadelphia, PA.
Tumor Type: Hodgkin's Lymphoma diagnosed September of 1994.
Treatment: Spleenectomy in October 1994 (to stop metastases), radiation
10/94-1/95. Remission for five months. Came out of remission in June
1995 and underwent 10 months of chemo through March 1996.
Photo Credit: Thomas Jefferson University.

WE MAKE PLANS AND GOD LAUGHS

"I had this well planned-out life. I was going to be a lawyer, have a nice house and a nice car. On September 5, 1994, everything changed."

Christopher Dezzi, now 27, was a senior in college when a minor complaint of a swollen gland in his neck lead to a biopsy and diagnosis of Hodgkin's disease.

"I was stunned—I was in total disbelief that something like this could happen to me at my age," Chris remembers. A week later, Chris underwent a spleenectomy, forcing him to leave school and begin daily radiation. "One of the hardest parts of leaving school was knowing that I wouldn't graduate with my friends eight months later."

Following radiation therapy, Chris remained in remission for five months. He then experienced a recurrence, for which he underwent nearly a year of chemotherapy.

"Before I was diagnosed, I was undefined," Chris reports. "I was unsure of who I was, of my abilities and what role I could play in this world. I left the cancer experience knowing exactly who I was, who my friends were and with a knowledge of what I was supposed to do with my life."

His new life's ambition centered on starting and running a successful business. Chris and his mother founded the Dezzi Group, a business and political consulting agency that services government and private industry in the Philadelphia area.

"My job helps define me as a person and it also gives me the opportunity to help a lot more people," Chris remarked. "I push myself pretty hard to achieve more things, which may stem from the fear that I might not be around long enough to achieve everything I'd like to."

With a successful business underway and his health in check, his near-term goals are to complete his Master's and Doctorate degrees and get married. Five years into his current remission, Chris is also a frequent traveler, citing it as a way to celebrate his life. He also pays close attention to his health through regular diet and exercise.

While he's very driven and goal-oriented, Chris isn't as serious as his demeanor may project. "When all's said and done, I want to have accomplished something," he said. "I can't really tell you what it is, because I don't think I know what it is yet. But I still want to have fun."

While in hot pursuit of his future goals, he has no regrets about his past. "If I had to do it all over again, I wouldn't change a thing," he remarked. "Cancer made me realize that life is too short and, as a result, I now approach every situation as an opportunity to meet new people and grow. I'm a lot stronger for having gone through this experience."

According to Chris, a family friend often quoted a Yiddish saying that Chris didn't fully appreciate until he got sick. "He used to say, 'we make plans and God laughs.' Not only do I now know what he meant, I also realize that the phrase fits my life to a tee."

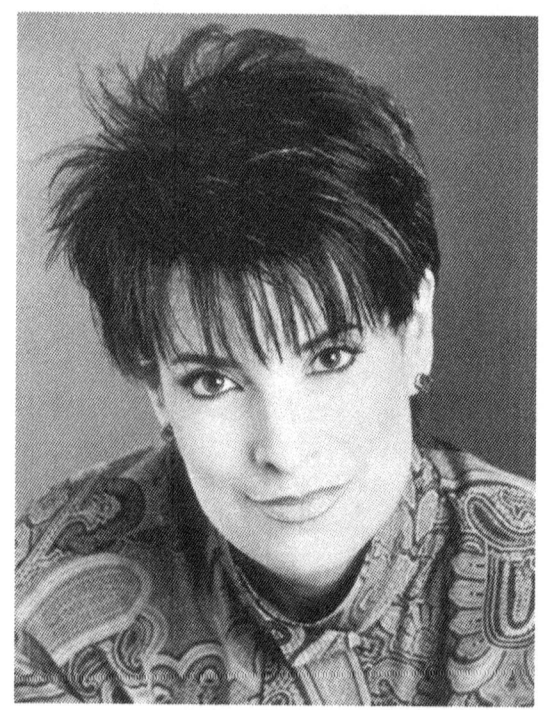

Selma Schimmel, 46

Single.

Selma is the founder and president of a national cancer communication support and advocacy organization called Vital Options. Selma hosts the radio show "Cancer Talk" that reaches nearly 400,000 listeners each week, now in its fifth year. It's been expanded to Europe and is Internet accessible. She has also written a book by the same name. To find the station nearest you that carries the show, visit the website at vitaloptions.org or call 800-477-7666.

Born: Los Angeles, CA. Lives: Los Angeles, CA.

Tumor Type: Breast Cancer, 1983.

Treatment: Lumpectomy, radiation and chemotherapy.

Photo Credit—Buddy Rosenberg.

CANCER TALKS, BUT I TALK LOUDER

The National Coalition for Cancer Survivorship (NCCS) defines survivorship as "the time of diagnosis through the rest of life, no matter what stage of disease you're in." Selma Schimmel agrees.

"I absolutely subscribe to that," declared Selma Schimmel, breast cancer survivor and founder of Vital Options, the first cancer support organization on the radio and internet. "I even look at the people I loved who've died of cancer—like my mother—as survivors, by virtue of their attitude and what they did to fight the disease."

Selma was diagnosed with breast cancer just after her mother died of ovarian cancer; other close family members have had cancer as well. "I was the first person diagnosed in my family who didn't die from cancer," Selma said. "Early diagnosis and modern technology saved me."

When she was diagnosed in her 20s, Selma's father became not only her dad, but her mom, best friend and spiritual advisor. Selma asked her father, a liberal Orthodox Rabbi, about his perception of God and whether that had changed following her mother's death.

"I remember him saying to me, 'I love God. I don't like what's happening, but I love God,'" Selma remembers. "Despite what he was going through, I saw how steadfast my father was and that his relationship with God was unchanged, which was a great lesson for me. I realized that, while I didn't necessarily like what God was doing, it didn't change my relationship with Him."

Selma underwent a lumpectomy, chemotherapy and radiation. "I got through the treatments knowing that it would come to an end—that I wouldn't have to do this for the rest of my life," she explained. "I thought of it as a short-term investment in my long-term well-being."

At the time, she never imagined that she would transform her cancer experience into her life's work. "I became a national advocate because I wanted to take my diagnosis and do something positive with it, especially enable others to learn, like I had, how to integrate cancer into their lives and live side-by-side with it," Selma remarked.

Through Vital Options, she advises the newly diagnosed to allow themselves time to grieve following their diagnosis. "Cancer is a huge intruder in your life, so cut yourself some slack," she says. "You're probably going to feel that your body has betrayed you, and that can leave you feeling overwhelmed and powerless."

She adds, "While you have to deal with all of these emotions, you also need to step back and make your clinical decisions not based on emotion, but on clear thought. This is when it becomes important to separate your heart from your head."

In her advocacy work, she has set her sights on the world. "Cancer is a global problem, and the access and treatment issues are universal," Selma remarked. "My vision is to realize a time when state-of-the-art cancer diagnosis, treatment and comprehensive care is available to you no matter who you are, what type of cancer you have or where you live."

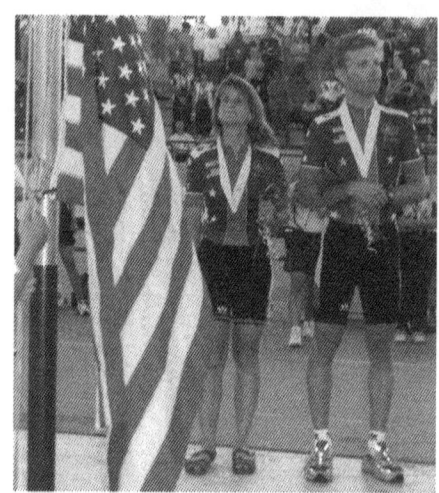

Cara Dunne-Yates, 30

Married 2 years with a daughter 8 months old.
Cara is a professional athlete and recently competed in the Sydney Para-Olympic games as a tandem cyclist in track sprinting. She was on the US Disabled Ski Team from 1982 through 1989.
Born: Chicago, Illinois. Live: Colorado Springs, Colorado.
Tumor Type: Bilateral Retinoblastoma (genetically based childhood eye cancer) diagnosed when she was 15 months old. At 23 she was diagnosed with Osteogenic Sarcoma in the right sinus. This year she was diagnosed with Leiomyosarcoma, with metastases to the liver and small intestines.
Treatment: Radiation and Chemotherapy followed by cryosurgery (freezing the tumors). First eye removed at age one, other eye removed at age five. Surgery for Osteogenic Sarcoma. Chemotherapy for Leiomyosarcoma.
Cara supports The National Association for Parents of the Visually Impaired, that can be reached at 1-800-562-6265. She also supports the Retinoblastoma Organization. She has also been awarded the Lance Armstrong Foundation's "Carpe Diem" award for "Spirit of Survivorship." Photo Credit: Unknown. At Para-Olympics, with professional cyclist Scott Evans.

FROM CHEMO TO KILO

At the age of 30, Cara Dunne-Yates is a mother with an undergraduate degree from Harvard, law degree from UCLA, and is a several-time medal winner in the U.S. Para-Olympic Games.

Talking with her, it almost comes as an aside that she is not only a cancer survivor, but is also blind.

Cara was diagnosed with a genetically based childhood cancer when she was just over a year old, necessitating removal of one eye and the second when she was five years old.

"In 1993, I was living in Utah and had been out of college for about six months," she remembers. "I was thinking about trying to find a guide to qualify for the 1994 Para-Olympics in Lillihammer, while I was working in a program that taught disabled kids how to ski."

After finding a lump on her cheekbone the size of a pecan, it was discovered that she had osteogenic sarcoma in her right sinus, a possible side effect of earlier radiation therapy as a child. She underwent chemotherapy and three surgeries, while remaining active in the Retinoblastoma Foundation.

She was only in her early '20s, and her friends had what they perceived as equally grave concerns. "I remember walking with a friend in Harvard Square after one of my surgeries, when she asked me how things were going," Cara said. "I remember telling her that things were pretty tough and she proceeded to report that she has had a tough time, too, being without a boyfriend for a few months." Cara laughs when she retells the story.

Nearly finished with her cycles of chemo, Cara had lunch with some close friends, most of whom also had some form of disability. "The place we wanted to go was closed and we were upset that we wouldn't be able to walk a half-mile to the nearest restaurant to get something to eat," she recounts. She said that it suddenly dawned on her that, with the assistance of her Seeing Eye dog, not only could she walk, but she could run to get the lunch and bring it back to her friends.

"I remember running and thinking that I can walk, and I can run, and my arms and legs still work," Cara remarked. "I remember at that moment thinking, "Maybe I'm going to make it.""

Throughout her life, Cara has been constantly reminded that her life is a work in progress. "After racing with the U.S. Disabled Ski Team for most of my teenage years, I was giving motivational speeches, thinking that the tough stuff was all behind me—that I had gone through everything I was going to go through," Cara remembers.

"Now I know that you'll never overcome everything you're going to have to overcome," she continued. "You're always in a state of working towards something and getting through something. That's why it's important to enjoy every day and try to find good memories in seemingly trivial moments, instead of aspiring to do something that may never really happen."

Cara won a silver medal in Atlanta in the 1996 Para-Olympics in the one-kilometer time trial and calls her experience "from chemo to kilo."

She is now undergoing chemotherapy for her third cancer, Leiomyosarcoma, recently won the Lance Armstrong Foundation's "Carpe Diem" award for "Spirit of Survivorship."

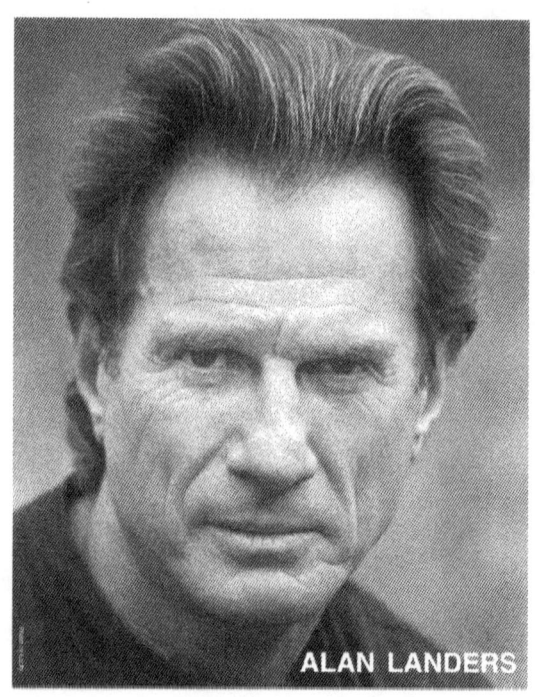

Alan Landers, 59

Single, no children.

Alan is the former Winston Man cigarette model. He is also an acting teacher, and was an actor and model. He is working on his autobiography "Kicking Butts."

Born: Brooklyn, NY (Flatbush). Lives: Fort Lauderdale, FL

Tumor Type: Bronchial carcinoma diagnosed February 1988 and Non-Small Cell diagnosed January 1993.

Treatment: Two lobes of the right lung removed (1988), one lobe of the left lung removed (1993).

Alan can be reached for public speaking engagements through his website, www.winstonman.com or by email at WINSTONMAN1@webtv.net or by phone at 954.731.3017

Photo Credit: Unknown. Just before second lung cancer operation.

KICKING BUTTS

The former Winston Man diagnosed with lung cancer—how ironic is that? Not very, since, at the time, two Marlboro men had already succumbed to the disease.

"Even though my surgeon told me not to smoke for at least 10 days prior to my operation, the night before I was sitting in a waiting room watching TV and smoking a cigarette," remembers Alan Landers. "That's how truly addicting nicotine is."

Alan's lung cancer was discovered when he underwent a chest X-ray prior to a hernia operation. "I thought the first time around that I was going to die for sure, since everyone I knew who had lung cancer did. I just kept praying to God that I wouldn't die."

He was diagnosed with a tumor the size of a golf ball on his other lung four years later. While removing one lobe of his lung, the surgeons accidentally severed his vocal cord, rendering him speechless for over a year.

Four years later, Alan was testifying in Washington before a Senate hearing on an anti-smoking program for children, when "my chest went on fire." He was suffering hardening of the arteries—a residual effect of smoking—and needed to undergo double bypass surgery.

Now nearly 60, Alan has just finished five years of depositions, after filing a lawsuit against the tobacco industry. He is also touring Asia with the World Health Organization (WHO) for two years to help share his experiences with a culture in which children are often given cigarettes when they're very young to help curb their appetite.

"There, it's considered 'unmanly' if you don't smoke, so nonsmokers are made fun of," Alan shared. He cited WHO statistics predicting that, in China alone, one-third of the 300 million male smokers will die within the next 20 years.

What has being in the trenches with the tobacco industry taught him? "It's been a sort of spiritual awakening," he remarked. "With two bouts of lung cancer, a heart operation and now, very little breathing, I believe God has me here for a purpose."

He told a story of doing a presentation to young children in Southeast Asia and encouraging them to "go home and sit on your papa's lap and tell him not to smoke because you're afraid he's going to die and you need a father.'"

The next day, the father of one of the young boys in the audience drove four hours to Alan's presentation, during which he confessed that he was a heavy smoker, and that he was afraid he was going to die if he didn't quit. "It was wonderful to know that my message is getting through. It's sort of like being a missionary."

Alan, like many people, learned from his mistakes. "I'm a lot stronger personally after cancer than I was before," he said. "Fear comes from not knowing and it can take away your will. So, go the other way—keep exercising, eat well, educate yourself and do what your doctors tell you. Say, 'I'm going to live one day at a time and do the best I can.'"

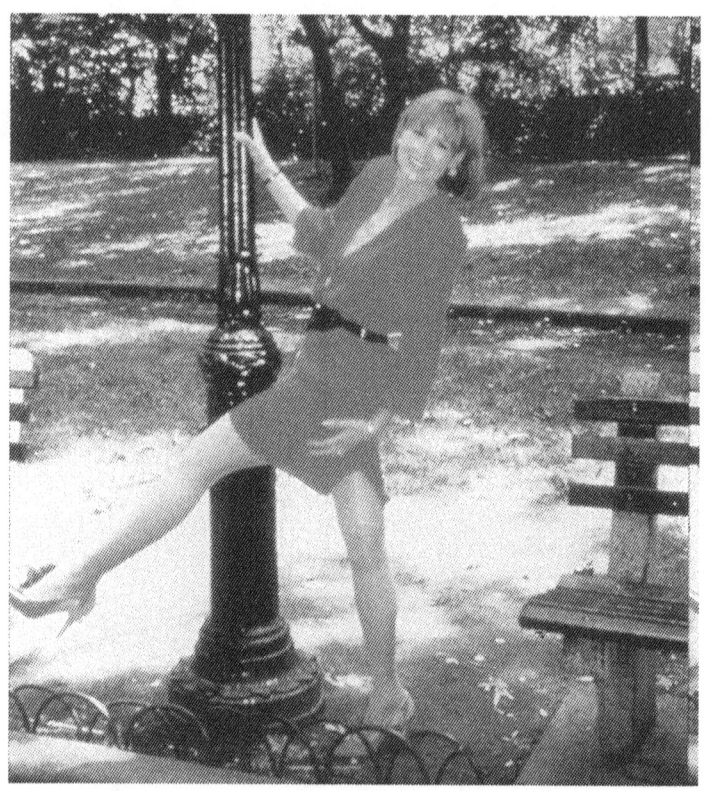

Ivy! Gunter, "30+"

Married "Many" years to Don.
Georgia Regional Sales Manager of a Gift and Home Accessory Company and author of the autobiography "On the Ragged Edge...of Drop Dead Gorgeous."
Born: Oak Ridge Tennessee; Live: Atlanta, GA.
Tumor Type: Osteogenic (bone) sarcoma, diagnosed March 31, 1980.
Treatment: Surgery and Chemotherapy.
Ivy! Can be contacted through "Speakers & Entertainment" Agent Richard Secotti at 914.271.5825 for speaking engagements.
Photo Credit: Unknown. Back in New York City, the capital of modeling.

FROM SUPERMODEL TO SUPERWOMAN

"When I was in the hospital, a prosthetic salesman came in to visit me and told me, 'There's going to be no more Calvin Klein tight jeans, no more high heels and no more straight skirts. I threw him out of my room.'"

These are the words of supermodel Ivy! Gunter, who lost her leg to cancer 20 years ago. My doctor told me, 'You can either die with two legs or you can live with one.'"

Ivy! experienced swelling in her leg, which she attributed to an injury. Before each photography shoot, the model immersed herself in a hot tub to relieve the pain. "In the beginning, I was in such denial because I was a model with one of the largest agencies in New York," she said. "I didn't want anything to burst my bubble."

X-rays diagnosed her tumor, which was encased on the back of her leg, preventing it from metastasizing. "Four days later, the amputation was performed above my knee, and it didn't even sink in that it was cancer until I heard the part about the chemotherapy," Ivy! explained.

Ivy! said that when she woke up following the surgery, her leg was gone. "When I woke up and I saw this empty space on the bed I thought 'Wow, they really did it.' For the first time in six months, I thanked God that there was no more pain," she said. During this time, when she had the visit from the prosthetics salesman, her business agent also left her. However, the good news offset the bad—following chemotherapy, her doctor told her she had a 98 percent chance of survival.

For months later, sporting a prosthesis that she designed herself, Ivy! participated in a photo shoot for *Atlanta* magazine and continued her modeling career, which was unheard of at that time. "I was bald as a cue ball, which was pretty funny since the movie, "Star Trek: The Motion Picture," had just come out, with the bald character played by the model Persis Khambatta.

She continued modeling with a new assortment of five wigs of varying colors. "It was all very theatrical," Ivy! remembers. "I scared the hell out of everyone when I walked in for an audition."

Over the past 20 years, she has continued to model, is a regular speaker at National Cancer Survivorship Day and learned to ski with the National Handicap Sports Association. "I met this guy who was a below-the-knee amputee and he double-dog-dared me to get out on the mountain," Ivy! recounts. "While I looked like a million bucks—bright yellow jacket, hot pink lipstick and perfectly polished nails—I wasn't a pretty sight when I ended up 50 yards away from my skis. But I didn't feel like I had a handicap because everyone is equal on the mountain: you all have to get to the bottom."

Ivy! has also become certified as a group and personal adapted fitness instructor for physically challenged people. "I'm very proud of this accomplishment. I want to help anyone with physical limitations—whether asthma, obesity or some other condition—to have a healthier lifestyle," she remarked. Her next event is a 60 mile walk over three days for breast cancer.

During her experience with cancer, her relationship with her friends has changed from superficial to intimate. "Many of them call me to ask if I'd talk with another friend of theirs who has been diagnosed with cancer," Ivy! reports. "I tell their friends to get back to work and get involved in something outside of themselves and chemotherapy—do something you can control."

Down deep, Ivy! truly believes she is a survivor. "When people ask me what I did to triumph over cancer, I tell them I'm as stubborn as hell," she muses. "I believe I have the inner strength to get through anything—job changes, life changes, you name it. I've had cancer threaten my life and I've been through fear and pain, but now I feel like a million dollars."

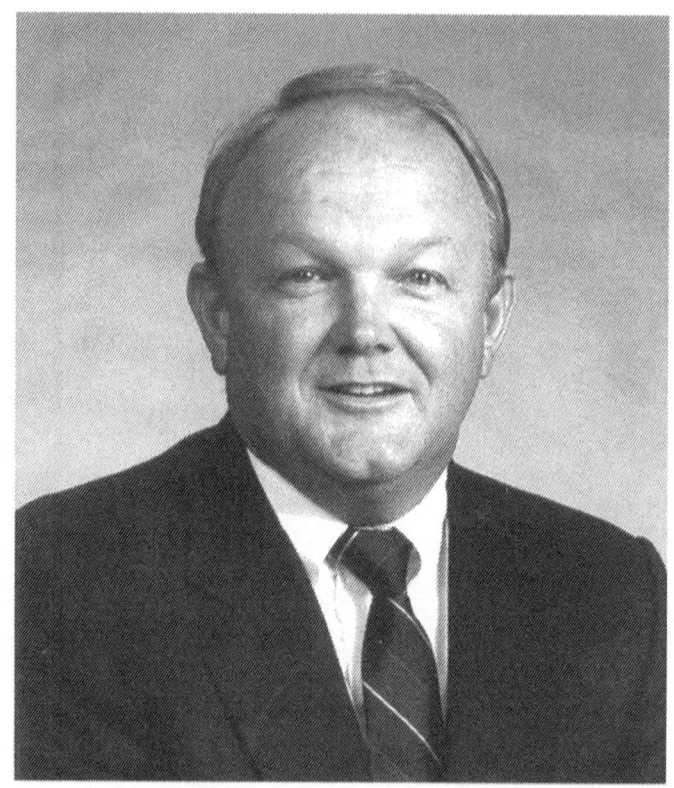

Tom Amick, 57

Married 6 years to Lisa; daughters Lauryn and Christine. Sons Bill and Brad from first marriage.
President of Ortho Biotech, Europe.
Born: Mebane, North Carolina; Live: London, United Kingdom.
Tumor Type: Teratoma (testicular), diagnosed 1993.
Treatment: Surgery.
Photo Credit: Ortho Biotech

DETERMINATION!!

When his cancer diagnosis was handed down, his thoughts were consumed as much with his psychological approach to the disease as with the medical path that would be undertaken.

"My life changed at the time of my diagnosis," expressed Tom Amick, a 57-year-old testicular cancer survivor. "From the very start, I thought about how I was going to beat this disease."

His thinking paid off. After successful surgery to remove his tumor, Tom began to live life to the fullest, perhaps for the first time. "I believe that everything happens for a reason, and my diagnosis was a real wake-up call to me," he remarked. "I decided that I didn't want to miss a thing in my life, and I wanted to be the very best I could be in everything I did."

Apparently, he is succeeding in meeting that goal. Since his diagnosis, he has remarried and had two children, and has been awarded six promotions to senior management with one of the world's largest health care companies. "I enjoy everything now, and there are no bad days," he said.

His competitive spirit served him well during his cancer experience, and is reflected into the sage advice he offers others who are recently diagnosed. "Go into this determined to win and don't ever give up. Having a positive attitude pays big dividends."

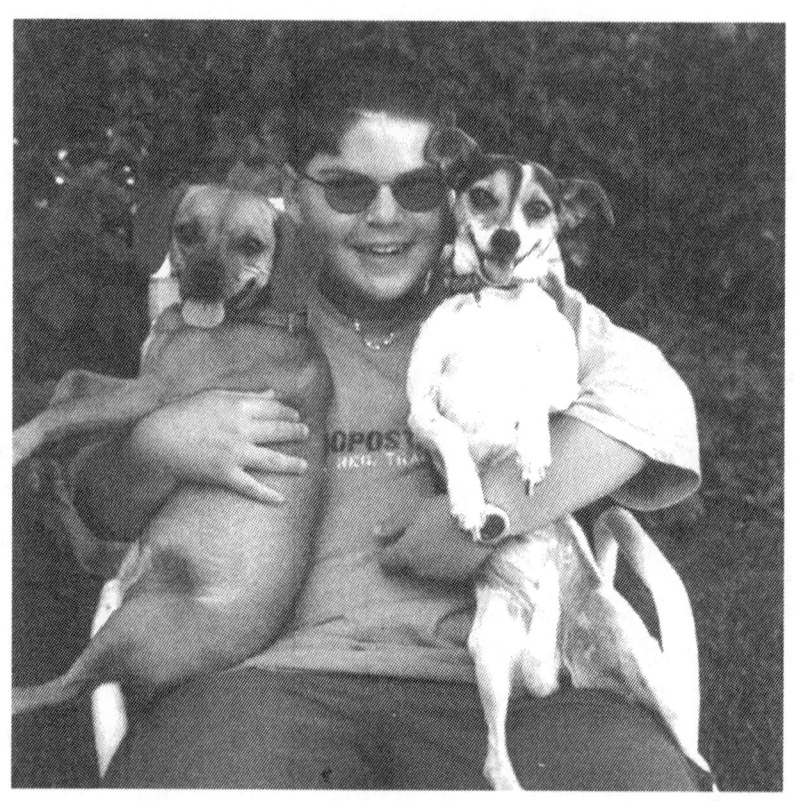

Kyle Benetz, 12

Single, "Of Course".
Seventh Grade Student.
Born: Rockledge, PA; Live: Rockledge, PA.
Tumor Type: Brain Cancer diagnosed 1990.
Treatment: Chemotherapy and Surgeries.
Photo Credit: Connie Benetz.

JUST A REGULAR KID

After 10 surgeries, countless rounds of chemotherapy and numerous seizures, 12-year-old Kyle Benetz calls himself a "typical" kid.

"Sure, there are some things I can't do, but I think I'm a little stronger because I've had so many surgeries and am still alive," he remarked. His mother also attributes his strength to his positive attitude and high threshold for pain.

Kyle was not yet three years old when he had severe headaches that lasted for six months. A CT scan determined that he had a large tumor in the center of the brain. He began more than a year of chemotherapy and surgeries, many of them high risk. During this time, he suffered a hernia from the severe vomiting caused by his chemotherapy, and experienced seizures as the tumor continued to grow and press on his brain stem.

In 1992, his tumor finally stopped growing and, as subsequent surgeries removed 90 percent of the tumor, his seizures stopped. Kyle is now considered in remission, undergoing no treatment other regular check-ups.

Kyle is very relaxed about discussing his challenging years, particularly when talking to other kids diagnosed with cancer. "Just deal with the pain. Try to keep up with everything and do your best. Just try not to think that you have whatever you have and just think that you're a typical person."

Part of being a "typical" pre-teenager for Kyle now involves trips to the Jersey shore in the summer, where he plays miniature golf, as well as a routine staple of video games, hanging out with his friends and watching TV.

"All the doctors said that Kyle's definitely an exception," his mom reports. "He tolerated the surgeries and has recovered at a very rapid rate with no side effects, no problems and no follow-up treatments."

In Kyle's words, "I'm just a regular kid!"

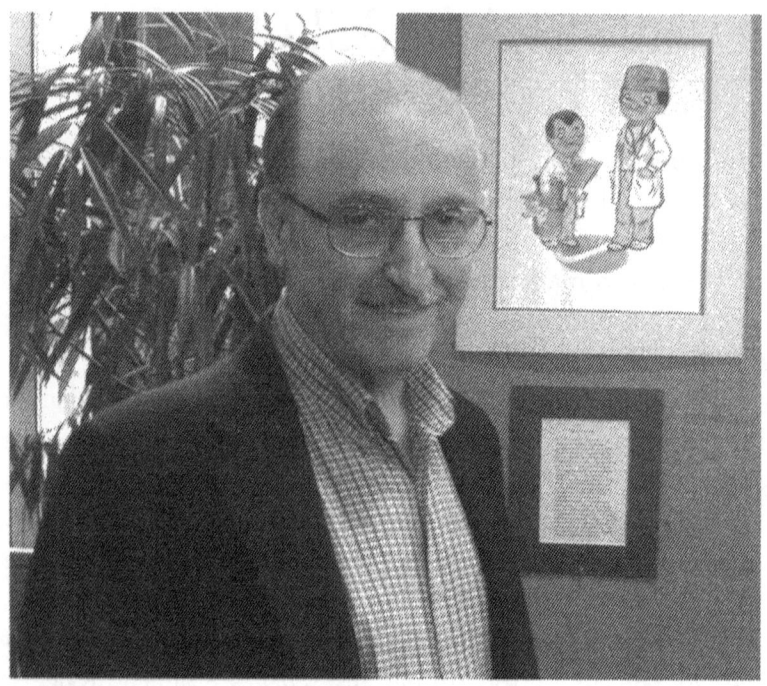

Sal Acerba, 73

Married 38 years with three children and two grandchildren.
Illustrator and commercial artist.
Born: Philadelphia, PA; Live: Blackwood, NJ.
Tumor Type: Rectal cancer diagnosed 1997.
Treatment: Radiation and Chemotherapy followed by surgery to remove a foot of colon, appendix and gall bladder.
Sal drew the Campbell's Soup Kids and other food labels since the 1950's. He also drew for many companies as a freelance illustrator (including the Franklin Mint) and as a medical illustrator for surgical equipment companies.
Photo Credit: Thomas Jefferson University Hospital at National Cancer Survivor's Day event.

NEVER TOO LATE

A cloudy family history of cancer doesn't mean that the diagnosis rains on your parade.

"Although cancer runs in my family, I still couldn't believe my diagnosis," remarked Sal Acerba, a 73-year-old illustrator and commercial artist, whose mother, father, brother and three sisters have succumbed to the disease.

Once he overcame the initial shock, Sal learned to deal with his fate. "While I initially didn't take the news too well, I quickly got over it and got on with what I needed to do," he said.

This entailed radiation and chemotherapy to attack his rectal cancer and a spot on his liver, followed by surgery to remove a large portion of his colon, appendix and gallbladder. "Even during treatment I was confident in the outcome. I got sleepy and only a little nauseous. Once I got the hiccups for two days. But I didn't let cancer beat me down."

Following successful treatment, he returned to his trade, which has become significantly computer-based in recent years. During his career, Sal drew the widely known Campbell's Soup Kids illustrations, along with other consumer and medical artwork.

"At the age of 70, I became curious about how computer-generated graphics are done, so I bought a computer and took some classes at our local college," Sal said. "I spend a good bit of time on it and it's kind of fun. I'm keeping busy that way between painting and working on the computer."

It's no secret that cancer changes people; unfortunately, it's not widely recognized that the changes can be for the better. In addition to honing his professional skills, Sal has also learned to relax more. "My wife and I are finally taking vacations. We like to exercise, and I walk everyday, stopping afterwards for a cup of coffee. It's something that I really look forward to and have made a lot of new friends."

Sal now tells his friends who have been recently diagnosed that cancer survival is all in how you approach it. "I know what they're feeling and I tell them I came through with flying colors. A good attitude about the whole thing and a strong belief in the power of prayer is what pulled me through."

He added that it's important to dismiss the outdated stereotypes the disease carries. "I saw a character on a TV soap opera who was diagnosed with cancer and the impression they gave on that show was that it's the end of the rope, like she'll die tomorrow. That's a terrible image."

Sal wastes no time in noting that, as a cancer survivor in his 70s, he's taking vacations, learning about computers, exercising, beginning to play golf, and he is now painting family portraits.

"Cancer isn't going to slow me down," he reports. "At my most recent doctor visit, I was given a clean bill of health and told to go out and celebrate. I was speechless. If I had tried to open my mouth, I would have broken down."

Cancer has taught Sal that you're never too old to stop learning. "Cancer changes your life, and you can't get away from that. But I used to be hesitant about things and now I'm not. I try not to let anything hold me back." Sal is happy to report that after having a defibrillator implanted for a heart problem that he is still doing well. "I am truly blessed".

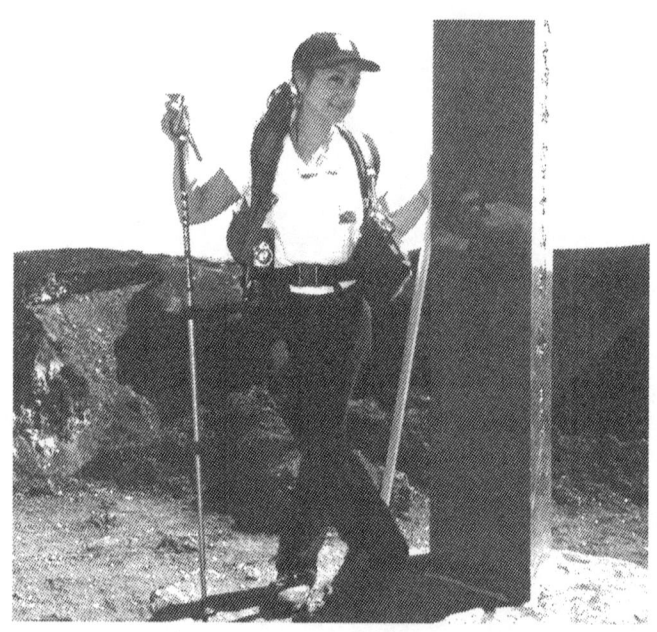

Cathy Masamitsu, 47

Single.

Cathy is a television producer and reporter for the "Home" show. Cathy is the first person to have been filmed during her treatments for television. Tens of thousands of copies of the 1989 taping have seen distributed. She is an ordained deacon and elder in the Presbyterian Church.

Born: Chicago, IL "Go Cubs!"; Lives: Los Angeles, CA

Tumor Type: Breast Cancer, twice, diagnosed 1986 and a recurrence in 1989. Treatment: Lumpectomy with follow-up radiation therapy and a mastectomy with reconstruction in 1989.

Cathy and nine other professional breast cancer survivors coauthored "BREAST CANCER? LET ME CHECK MY SCHEDULE!" with all author proceeds directed to breast cancer education and advocacy groups. Photo Credit: Vicki Smith. At the summit of Mt. Fuji (Japan) for the Breast Cancer Fund.

BREAST CANCER?
LET ME CHECK MY SCHEDULE!

The good news is that the second time you go through cancer, you know what to expect. That's also the bad news.

"I think second diagnosis is a really important thing to deal with because it is a major terror for people who have had cancer before," explained Cathy Masamitsu, a two-time breast cancer survivor. "The first time, I was 32 and I didn't even know what a mammogram was. The second time, I thought I knew everything, but I soon learned that facing recurrence was a whole new ball of wax."

A producer and reporter for TV's "Home" show, Cathy allowed live television cameras to document her treatments—a network first. "The power of the media is astonishing. Even now, more than a decade later, people remember watching my story and seek me out to talk about their diagnosis," she reported. "I decided early on in the battle, even before my surgery, I was going to share something deeply personal in a very public way. It changed my life, but I don't regret it."

Cathy commented on the "sorority" that bonds women with breast cancer to each other and the public at large. "The remarkable thing about cancer in general and breast cancer in particular is that there's an astounding percentage of women who say 'when I get past this, I want to do something to make it easier for somebody else'."

Cathy's experiences are chronicled in her co-authored book, *"Breast Cancer, Let me Check My Schedule"*. She said that many of the women interviewed for the book shared a common theme—that they attacked cancer as they would approach a difficult assignment in the workplace. "After recovering from the initial shock of diagnosis, we thought—'I don't want to do this, but if I MUST, I'm going to do it WELL!'—that helped us get through it."

Cathy says that cancer gave her a new perspective that gave clarity to her priorities in life. "Before cancer, traveling was always something I was going to get around to 'someday'—but now I don't put things off." She started planning her first big vacation from her hospital bed, recovering from lumpectomy surgery. In the past decade, Cathy has traveled all over the world. Cathy recently climbed to the summit of Mt. Fuji, Japan, raising thousands of dollars for research for The Breast Cancer Fund— "Mt. Fuji was the greatest physical challenge I've undertaken in the war against this disease," she said proudly.

In the scheme of her life, cancer has been the great equalizer. "Sure, it was the worst crisis I've ever experienced. I was never so afraid in my life," Cathy remarked. "But it's also given me the blessing of doing something that was exactly what God wanted me to do—I was never more connected with Him."

Cathy is pleased that she shared her experience. "The public continues to benefit from our change in attitude about the disease in terms of research and early detection, and all cancers have benefited from the recognition that support groups are an important part of the healing process," she expressed. "Support groups are one of the most important things that someone fighting cancer can do for themselves," Cathy added.

A journalist by trade, there are many quotes that Cathy finds relevant to her own experiences. Among them is one from Frank Lloyd Wright suggesting that the project you should be most excited about is your next one. Another is that you haven't really lived until you've almost died, and that "for those who have fought for it, life has a flavor that the protected will never know."

A quote of her own is from a television interview in which Cathy was asked what it was like to be cancer-free. "I answered, 'I will know that on the day they find a cure for this disease. I refuse to celebrate my survivorship until that day, because until then, none of us is truly cancer-free. I'm convinced that they will find a cure in our lifetime'."

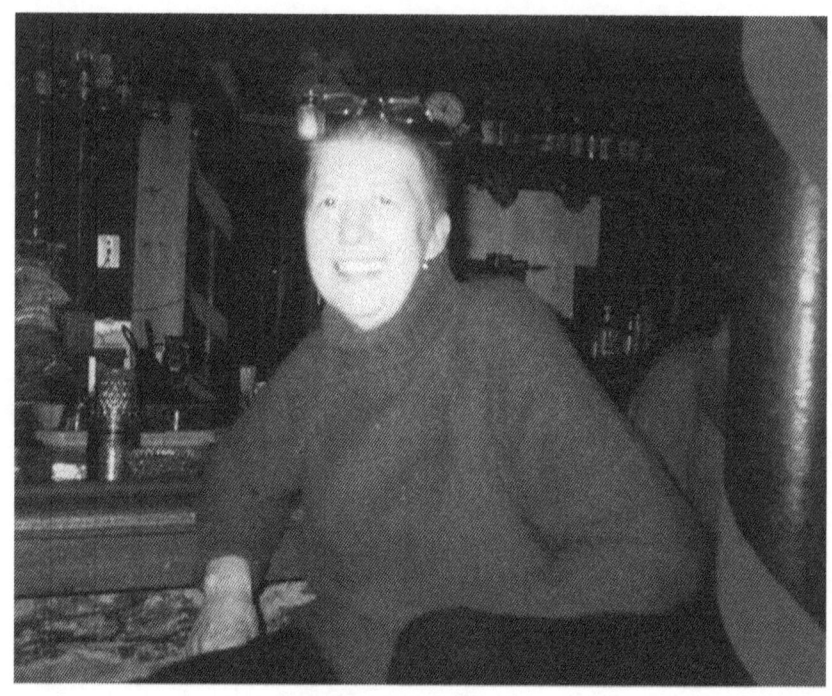

Nancy Blackwell, 60

Single, two kids: Jay (34) and Robin (39).
Chef, Owner and Manager of 150 year old Blackwell's National Hotel in Frenchtown, NJ.
Born: Ringoes, NJ; Live: Frenchtown, NJ.
Tumor Type: Small Cell Lung Cancer with local metastases, diagnosed July 1999.
Treatment: Radiation and Chemotherapy.
Photo Credit: Jennifer Safino.

SHE FIRED HER DOCTOR

A 60-year-old lung cancer survivor, Nan is the owner and manager of the historic Blackwell's National Hotel in Frenchtown, New Jersey, and an avid antique restorer.

"While I was terrified when I went in for my biopsy, I had a good attitude about wanting to beat the cancer right from the outset," she said. "In addition to my mental attitude, I was greatly consoled by the fact that medicine has advanced so quickly and there were many more options available to me than would have been in the past."

Nan's diagnosis came after months of feeling tired. "My doctor originally thought I had Lyme disease because I spend a lot of time with my dogs in the woods. My arms were so weak that I couldn't even chop vegetables," she said. Nan also experienced two bouts of pneumonia, for which she was prescribed antibiotics. "I was frustrated and felt like I was up against a brick wall and getting nowhere, because I wasn't being treated correctly," she added. So she fired her doctor.

Through a friend's father, who was a doctor, Nan was referred to an internist who did blood work and confirmed that she didn't have Lyme disease. "She sent me for an X-ray and identified the tumor right away. Thankfully, I had the sense to switch doctors or it could have been months before I was finally diagnosed," she remarked.

Following successful chemotherapy and radiation, Nan has resumed her active lifestyle. She is currently refurbishing the hotel, and preparing to move to a farm across the Delaware River with her boyfriend of 16 years, Tom. Their plans include expanding the farmhouse and adding a woodworking shop so that Nan can continue to refinish all of her own furniture and restore antiques, as well as craft the trim and woodwork for the house.

"Maybe some day I'll retire," she mused. "When I was younger and before my diagnosis, I used to take life for granted. But now I value my time more than ever before."

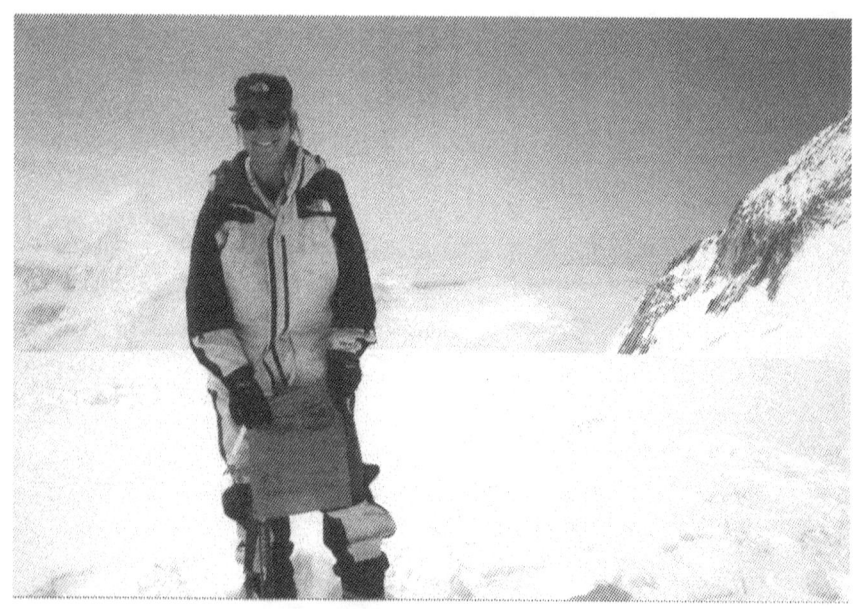

Mary Ann Castimore, 47

Married 4 years to John G. Lent.
Mountain climber and owner of the Beaverbrook Christmas Tree Farm in Augusta, NJ.
Born: Newton, NJ; Live: Augusta, NJ.
Tumor Type: Breast Cancer, diagnosed June 1986. Metastases to sternum and lungs February 1995.
Treatment: Modified radical mastectomy and Tamoxifen treatment until October 2000.
Mary Ann does a great deal of work for the Breast Cancer Fund (www.breastcancerfund.org), and the video of her climbs, called "Climb Against The Odds" can be purchased from them toll free at 866-760-8223.
Photo Credit: Unknown. Mary Ann on Mount McKinley at 14,200 feet.

ONE STEP AT A TIME

Ironically, it was altitude sickness, not cancer, that held Mary Ann back from reaching the summit of Mount McKinley in Alaska.

"It's an exhilarating experience to stand on top of a mountain and just look below you and see all the beauty," Mary Ann describes. "When you come down and see a picture of that mountain, you can rightfully say, 'that's my mountain,' because you stood on top of it."

Originally diagnosed with breast cancer in 1986, Mary Ann was past the "magic five-year mark" signifying a cure, when she woke up nine years later with a crushing pain in her chest.

At the time, she was leaving for a ski trip, so her doctor told her to call him if it still hurt when she returned. "I skied every day and lay in absolute agony at night," Mary Ann remembers.

Following her return, bone and CT scans confirmed a fractured sternum, caused by a malignant bone tumor. The cancer had also spread to her lungs. "The shock was, I went to bed thinking I was cured, and I awoke the next morning at stage four and there wasn't anything in-between."

"My physician determined that my tumors were estrogen-receptive, so they put me on Tamoxifen, which I was able to stop in October of 2000," she said. "I'm considered stable, which means no shrinkage, but no growth."

Now an avid mountain climber, Mary Ann has already climbed to the highest points in 49 states, and her husband has climbed all 50. "I climbed to 19,200 feet on McKinley in Alaska, so I've made 49 and 9/10. We've climbed Kilimanjaro, the highest point in the continent of Africa, at over 19,000 feet," she explained.

"It's very important for me to stand on top of Mt. McKinley just to convey that message of hope to breast cancer survivors and metastatic cancer survivors to never, never, ever give up hope," Mary Ann said. "Last time I got turned away 1000 feet from the summit it wasn't because of cancer, but due to a bout with altitude sickness."

She also ran a half-marathon of 13 miles in Tanzania, with her husband, who is an accomplished marathoner. Mary Ann climbed Mt. Fuji in Japan for the Breast Cancer Fund, with 200 Japanese women and 70 Americans.

Cancer has shown her the importance of appreciating what she has, more than what she doesn't. "It may sound strange to say, but I have never been happier in my life than I am now," she remarked. "I'd be happier if I didn't have to deal with cancer, but maybe that's what it took for me to appreciate what I have."

When asked if climbing mountains is like fighting cancer, Mary Ann says that both are taken one step at a time, but adds two differences. "Cancer is a terrible thing. Climbing mountains is a happy thing. Mountain climbing is a choice, while cancer is not. Besides, mountain climbing is easier than public speaking."

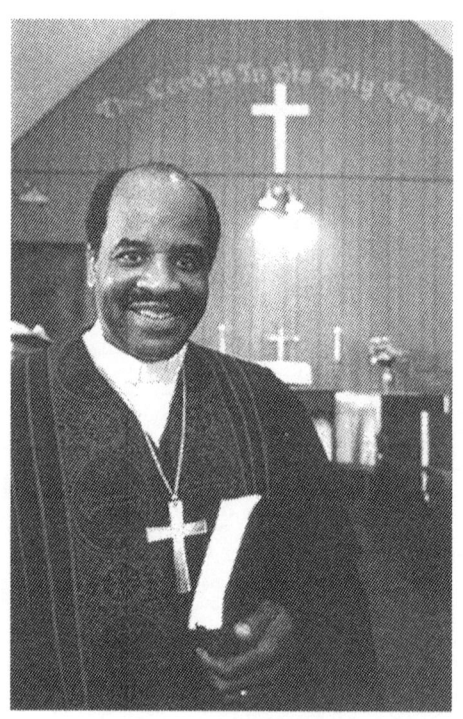

Dr. Michael Jerome Posey, 52

Married 19 years to Dr. Monica J. Posey, with two children 31 and 33, and three step-children.

Michael is pastor of the St. Paul AME Zion Church in Covenant, Kentucky, and was an Engineer at Procter and Gamble before taking early retirement. He is also a part time adjunct assistant professor at the University of Cincinnati in Mechanical Engineering Technology.

Born: Cincinnati, OH. Lives: Cincinnati, OH

Tumor Type: Third Stage Bile Duct Cancer without metastases diagnosed September 9, 1999.

Treatment: Surgery, Chemotherapy and Radiation.

Photo Credit—Lisa Ventre

UNCONDITIONAL FAITH IN GOD

Cancer hasn't changed him that much. Michael Posey always lived his life by the philosophy that there may not always be a tomorrow.

This engineer, pastor and seventh degree Black Belt in Tang Soo Do—and now cancer survivor—said, "I've always lived by the philosophy that if I had only three months to live, how would I choose to spend my time?"

After a diagnosis of bile duct cancer, he was given a 25 percent chance of surviving five years. Following, Michael underwent a nine-hour surgery in which he had a portion of his pancreas, intestines, stomach and bile duct removed. As if that wasn't enough, a surgical error left his arm partly paralyzed and a sponge was left in after the surgery, requiring another procedure to remove it.

During his paralysis, he completed his Doctoral dissertation, typing with his opposite hand. "I didn't want to die and not complete my dissertation, so it helped keep me motivated." Michael defended his dissertation on May 4, 2000—eight months after diagnosis—and won a "most outstanding doctoral student of the year" award. He also has Master's Degrees in business and theology.

Michael's other notable accomplishments include the completion of a seventh-degree black belt in Tang Soo Do—the martial art practiced by Actor Chuck Norris—after 30 years of training. Michael attributes this as a factor in his successful healing, along with a much more disciplined diet of green tea, fruit and vegetables, and abstinence from foods with added chemicals and preservatives.

Since retiring, he has also become a full-time pastor, after practicing part-time for many years. Michael was recently selected by his Bishop as the most outstanding minister in his Episcopal area of 500 clergy members. He has performed a great deal of ministry in Northern Kentucky in financially disadvantaged areas. Local parishioners have suffered and identify with him. "I share and they are totally engaged," he adds.

"After cancer, I now have much better insight into the concept of unconditional trust in God, even when things don't work out the way you want," he reflects. "I'm not afraid to die because I've made peace with God and with myself. On the other hand, I'm not going to volunteer to cross over—I'm going to fight every step of the way." Michael laughs. He adds, "If your doctors give you only six months to live, always remember that they're not the final judge."

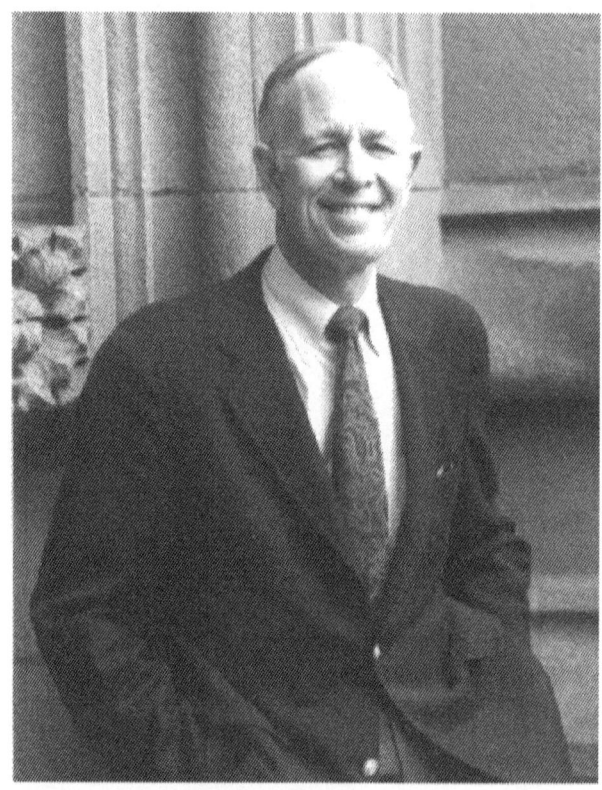

Dr. Robert Fagles, 66

Married 44 years with daughters Katya (35) and Nina (33).
Robert is the Arthur W. Marks class of 1919 Professor of Comparative Literature at Princeton University, and has taught there for forty years. His recent translation of the Greek epic Homer's Odyssey has met with great critical acclaim.
Born: Philadelphia, Pennsylvania. Live: Princeton, New Jersey.
Tumor Type: Breast cancer (1% of breast cancers are in men) diagnosed in the winter of 1992.
Treatment: Modified mastectomy March 12, 1992.
Photo Credit: Mary Cross

A PIECE OF GOOD LUCK

Cancer makes you contemplate your own mortality, and realize that life is a "profound and passionate thing," in the words of Oliver Wendell Holmes, Jr.,—and cancer survivor Dr. Robert Fagles.

Robert is a Professor of Comparative Literature at Princeton University, where he has taught for 40 years. From cancer, he has derived much more meaning than from any literary classic.

"Since I had never been seriously sick before, I had the typical reaction to my cancer diagnosis—a profound sense of dislocation, feeling unnerved and really not knowing what to think," Dr. Fagles remembers.

His breast cancer—which occurs in men only one percent of the time—was discovered after Robert complained of feeling sensitivity in his chest when it came in contact with his pocket pen. His physician immediately removed the tumor, followed by subsequent removal of additional tissue.

Robert's surgery was successful in eradicating the tumor and he now undergoes only routine annual checkups. His experience gave his life a new microfocus.

"I began to contemplate how precious life is, and began to value things moment- by-moment, more intensely and more vividly then I had before," he expressed. "I also counted my blessings and thanked my lucky stars that I was still around to do that. This contemplation of mortality has never left me since."

Ever since, Robert has continued to pursue his life's work with a passion, having recently translated the Greek epic Homer's "Odyssey" with great critical acclaim. He will soon address the formidable challenge of translating Virgil's "Aeneid".

Does he draw any parallels to his literary work and his own cancer experience? "Hanging out with things which are ancient Greek, I think you get the idea that life is not easy, that life is a question of struggle, but the struggle can be ennobling too," he remarked. "I'm still forming my knowledge of myself, and whether I'll ever accomplish that task, I don't really know. I wouldn't dream of hiding my experience—I'd like to share it with anyone who's interested."

What Robert immediately shares are three tips for newly diagnosed individuals: "Be with doctors whom you trust completely; value your partners, your children and your friends; and find a way of realizing—if you haven't already—how truly precious life itself really is."

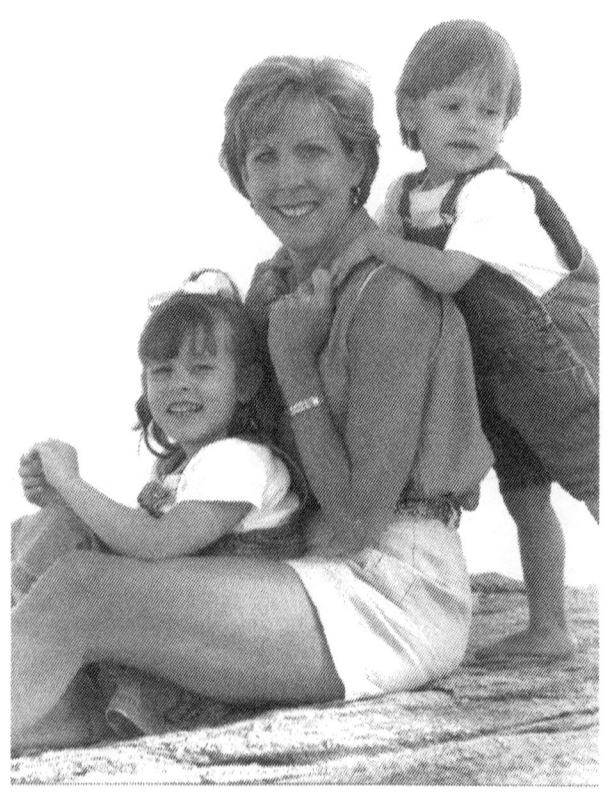

Kathy Giusti, 41

Married 10 years to Paul, children Nicole (5) and David (3).
President of the Multiple Myeloma Research Foundation (www.multiplemyeloma.org), a non-profit organization dedicated to raising awareness and funding research for Multiple Myeloma.
Born: Chestnut Hill, Pennsylvania; Live: New Canaan, CT.
Tumor Type: stage one Multiple Myeloma, diagnosed January 1996.
Treatment: Monitor disease, takes bone-density building drug to reduce the risk of fractures.
Photo Credit: Penny Millar.

A MOTHER'S LOVE

Once the highest ranking woman executive at a major pharmaceutical company, Kathy Giusti says that managing cancer is a lot like managing a business.

"First, you have to research and identify the best team, seek out and organize information and support, motivate your team and then let them know that you appreciate what they do for you," explained Kathy, a Harvard MBA and, now, president of the Multiple Myeloma Research Foundation.

She was diagnosed with Multiple Myeloma while undergoing a routine exam in preparing to have a second child. "My first thought was for my little girl," Kathy recalls. "She was only a year and a half old, and I kept thinking that I wouldn't live to see her enter kindergarten," since Multiple Myeloma has no known cure.

In true fashion, Kathy fought not only her cancer, but also continued her fight to have a second child. "Although my doctors were very skeptical, I underwent in vitro fertilization," she said. "The first procedure failed, but the second was successful. The day my son was born was the highest of highs—it really turned things around for me."

According to Kathy, following a cancer diagnosis, if you keep focused on what's important to you, you tend to think more about the goals than the disease. "You have to say to yourself, 'I'm going to keep trying, I'm going to keep fighting and I'm going to do my best.'

While Kathy loved the challenges of the business world, cancer stopped her in her tracks. "With my diagnosis, I realized that what I was most proud of wasn't my business success, but my family," she remarked.

Kathy left the company, and she and her twin sister founded the Multiple Myeloma Research Foundation in 1996. The organization now has an executive director, paid staff and 150 volunteers who dedicate their time to supporting patients, furthering clinical research and serving as advocates in Washington. The Foundation is now ranked in the top 10 percent of all healthcare nonprofit organizations.

True to her nature, Kathy poured all of her passion into her work, only to realize that, as in the corporate world, she needed to stop and smell the roses. "I'm much more patient and my life is more balanced now. I still work incredibly hard at the MMRF but make certain not to miss special moments with my family. I know how precious those moments are."

Now, Kathy's family is her primary focus. "The biggest challenge I have right now is just making sure my kids live a happy life and that our family's where it needs to be," she said. "When I ask my daughter what I do for a living, she says, 'Mommy helps sick people.' I work so hard to find a cure because I never want my children to look back and say that their mommy didn't fight."

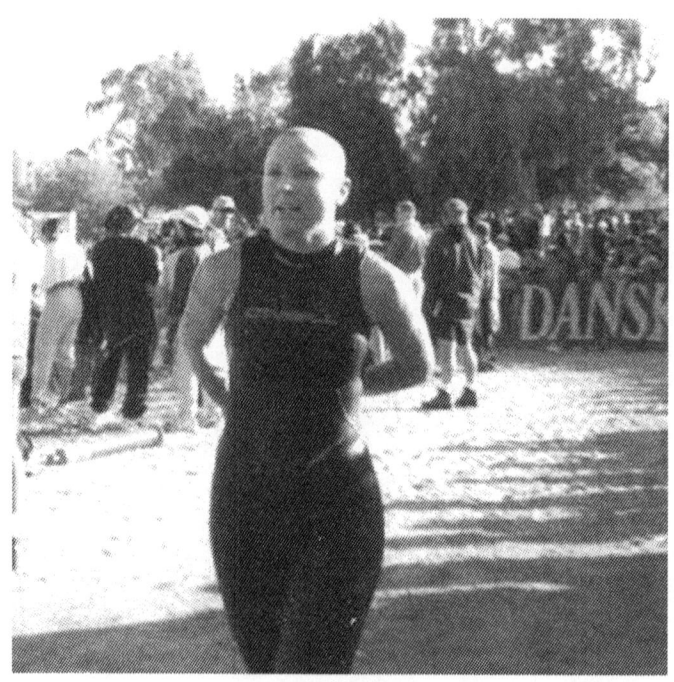

Kristin Bauersfeld, 31

Divorced.

User Interface Designer for Oracle, a major computer software company. "I help make software easy for people to use."

Born: Washington, DC; Live: Redwood City, CA.

Tumor Type: Breast Cancer (stage 2a) diagnosed April 1999.

Treatment: Radiation and Chemotherapy with Surgery (lumpectomy and the removal of two involved lymph nodes).

Kristin is involved in the "Team Survivor" Organization, a non-profit nationwide organization to provide exercise and health awareness to women in all stages of cancer. They provide many fitness activities and can be found on the web at www.teamsurvivor.org.

Photo Credit: Unknown—taken days after first chemotherapy treatment at her first triathlon.

THE EXCEPTION, NOT THE RULE

Kristin is by everyone's definition a "team survivor."

A year following her breast cancer diagnosis, she is an accomplished triathlete and competing equestrian. Kristin is also active in "Team Survivor," a national organization that supports women by helping them gain control over their cancer experience through preventive health and exercise.

"My whole life changed when I attended their first meeting," Kristin explained. "It was so amazing to listen to the stories of what some of the women in the group had been through—women who had bone marrow transplants and then six months later were doing a triathlon. They were incredibly inspiring and people I could relate to."

Kristin was diagnosed with breast cancer just after turning 30, six months after separating from her husband. She underwent radiation, chemotherapy and a lumpectomy with the removal of two lymph nodes. "This was a very big growth time for me," Kristin remembers.

She was supported by a strong network of friends and family, including her step-sister, Christine Clifford (see her interview), who had been diagnosed five years earlier, and her mother, who flew up to help her during her treatments.

Her friends were equally supportive and helped her evaluate the risks and benefits of the numerous potential treatment options. "It was a matter of trade-offs," Kristin reports. "It all came down to looking at what long term side affects I was willing to live with weighed against the potential success rates of each potential therapy."

She recalls having dinner with six very close friends to debate her options. "One of my really close friends was the last to open up," Kristin remembers. "She said, 'I think you should go for the treatment that is going to give you the best chance of survival that has the best track record at this point.' She said that this was my chance to be selfish, and that really made an impact on me and my decision."

As many patients find, chemotherapy left her with not as many horror stories to tell as she anticipated. "I had these visions of wasting away on a couch and feeling really bad, which is so counter to what I'm about," Kristin remarked. "I teach aerobic classes, I ride my horse, I run—I'm a very active person."

It's no surprise that she considers finding out about "Team Survivor" as one of the key turning points in her cancer experience—a discovery she made just prior to starting chemotherapy.

Kristin met with members of the organization two weeks into treatment. She decided to participate in the group's upcoming race as a walker, although she was running even after her recent lumpectomy.

"When I told one of the women that I could probably do the triathlon next year, she responded, 'You can do this now and you're going to.'" Kristin completed the triathlon—a half-mile swim, followed by a 12.2 mile bike race, and 13.2 mile run.

"That was an incredibly empowering experience, and made me realize how valuable exercise could be in fighting my cancer," Kristin said. "When I exercised, my body seemed to recover more quickly from the treatments. As a result, I stayed active through nearly my entire therapy through running, swimming and doing triathlons."

In the year following, she completed two similar triathlons, two "Olympic" events of twice the length and has signed up for her first "Iron Man" event—a 3 mile swim, followed by a 100 mile bike ride and 26.2 mile marathon run. Kristin also competes in a horseback riding event called "three-day evening," a competition over three days, now alternating one triathlon and one horse show every month.

"You can even take an experience like cancer and turn it around into something very meaningful," Kristin offered. "Cancer has given me a sense of empowerment, perspective, and the ability to inspire and motivate others who are going through similar experiences."

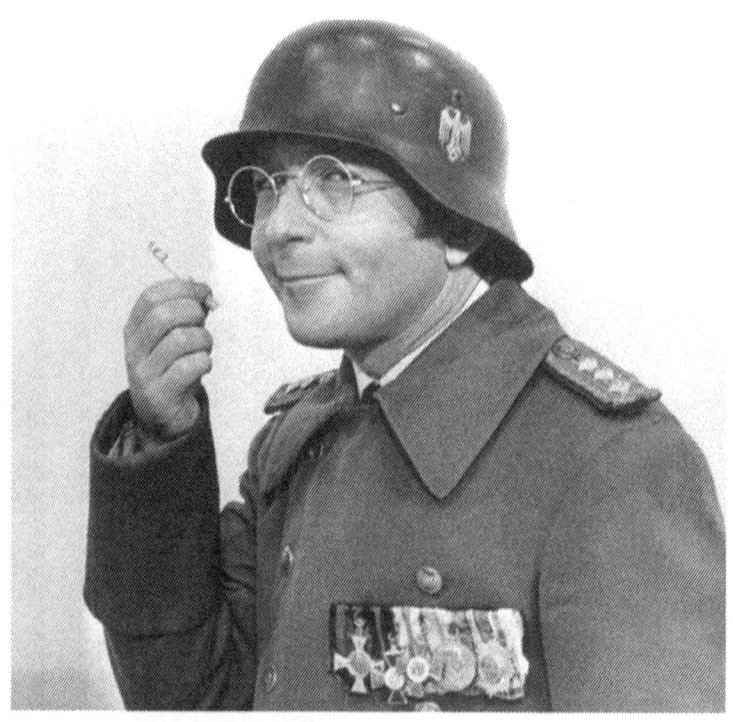

Arte Johnson, 71

Married 32 years to Gisela, no children.

Arte is a semi-retired actor and is best know for his roles on the 70's television comedy show "Laugh-In".

Born in Michigan. Lives: Los Angeles, CA.

Tumor Type: Non-Hodgkin's Lymphoma diagnosed 1997; Prostate Cancer diagnosed February 2001.

Treatment: Chemotherapy for Lymphoma; Radical Prostatectomy (surgical removal of Prostate) for Prostate cancer.

Arte supports the Leukemia and Lymphoma Society of America (on the web at http://l3.leukenia-lymphoma.org/hm-lls)

Photo Credit: NBC.

AIN'T LIFE WONDERFUL

When nationally renowned comedian Arte Johnson discovered he had cancer, he didn't want to immerse himself in medical textbooks. "I told my wife to go out and get me the funniest books she could find," he said.

Arte was working on Broadway when he discovered a swelling under one arm. "My friend and internist, Dr. Wilbur Schwartz, came backstage after my performance. When he found out about the underarm swelling it was he who insisted I see a physician who subsequently discovered a tumor in my lung."

The tumor was removed through an endoscopic procedure. While the tumor was benign, the surrounding lymph nodes were infected, necessitating him to undergo chemotherapy immediately for the Non-Hodgkin's Lymphoma. Even with a physician as a friend, Arte sees the most important factor in his survival as his wife Gisela. "Thank God she pushed me to get the thing looked at," he said.

"I feel magnificent," Arte purports. "I'm probably in better shape now than I've ever been because I'm actually taking better care of myself than I ever have before."

The chemo was debilitating for Arte, and he lost a role in a show he was seeking due to his illness. "Even on the worst days, I never lost sight of the fact that I was going to come out of this," he remembers. "I didn't read sad books and didn't want people coming around with bad stories. I didn't want to know about sadness."

He continued, "I've always thought of life as a fun thing, not something to really get crazy about. I just had to remind myself of that." Arte was also pleased to report that while he and Gisela traveled during his recovery, his hair stubble attracted fellow cancer survivors, who reveled in the fact that they hadn't curtailed their activities. However, Arte acknowledges the serious side. "I'm happy when I see people with a name using it as a platform to help others, like Michael J. Fox has done with Parkinson's disease."

He does feel fortunate to have been diagnosed in the midst of such swift medical advances. "There are discoveries being made every day, and everyone's got a shot at beating cancer," he offered. "You can't lose hope. It's not the end, and certainly not the end of the world." Four years after his lymphoma diagnosis, Arte became a "double-survivor", having beaten prostate cancer with the surgical removal of his prostate.

When he's not performing, Arte reads avidly and plays golf. He also sees movies to keep himself entertained. "There's no way I'm going to just sit and vegetate," Arte remarked. "Now I can enjoy the little things in life."

"We survivors are obligated to let people know that there is always that hope and that they should not give up. I was upset when I started to lose my hair from chemo, but I saw that the hair grows back."

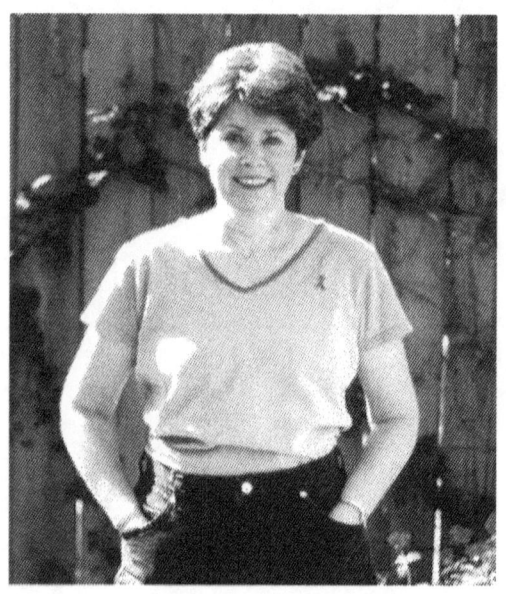

Pati Lanning, 49

Married 31 years to Roy, son (30) and daughter (24), plus a grandson. *Pati is a homemaker.*

Born: St. Paul MN. Lives: Harvey, LA

Tumor Type: Colon cancer diagnosed July 1998 "stage 2 to 3".

Treatment: Radiation, Chemotherapy, and eight inches of her colon was removed.

Pati supports the American Cancer Society, the Colon Cancer Alliance (CCA) and the EXTENSIVE list of services, support groups and online chat rooms at the Association of Cancer Online Resources, found at www.acor.org. She was interviewed in the July, 2000 "Better Homes and Gardens" magazine about her experiences and her quotes appear in Lorraine Johnston's book "Colon and Rectal Cancer: A Complete Guide for Patients and Families." (O'Reilly & Associates, Inc. Sebastopol, CA 1999)

Photo Credit: Roy Lanning. Taken in her prized garden.

VIKING WARRIOR WOMAN/STUBBORN SCOT

After her diagnosis of colon cancer, she surrounded herself with positive energy.

"That's the advice my surgeon gave me," Pati recalls. "He said, 'I don't care if you have to be rude, just get away from all of the negative people who tell you sad stories about how awful this is going to be.'"

Prior to her diagnosis, Pati had the classic symptoms of colon cancer, which was confirmed through colonoscopy and biopsy. "My awareness was pretty high—it was at a time when my mother had previously been diagnosed and Katie Couric's husband had just died from the disease," she said.

She took her diagnosis hard. "During the first three days, I just cried," Pati recalls. "Then one day I was praying, and this feeling just washed over me and I knew that everything was going to be okay."

She underwent radiation, surgery and nearly a year of chemotherapy. "When I read the package insert for the chemotherapy regimen, it didn't look good," Pati remarked. Despite nausea and fatigue, her doctors told her that she "sailed right through" her treatments. "Before treatment I steeled myself by dubbing myself the Viking Warrior Woman/Stubborn Scot based on my origin. How could I lose?"

Pati now volunteers with the Colon Cancer Alliance (CCA) www.CCAlliance.org as a buddy via email with the newly diagnosed, buddy chat coordinator and is active with CCA's newsletter and website. "I received tremendous support from people when I was diagnosed," Pati said. I was blessed to have such support of family, friends and online buddies and a wonderful group of doctors. I just couldn't have lucked out any better than I did. Now, I want to give something back."

In addition to her support group work, Pati is an avid gardener and makes her own paper by wetting, shredding and pressing used paper. "I have created two flower beds in my backyard, and feel really blessed that I was strong enough to get outside, dig up all that grass and put the plants in," Pati said. "When I'm out there working in the garden, it just hits me over and over again how wonderful it is to go out, soak up the sun and look at the butterflies."

She feels it's important to keep as busy as you can to distract yourself during treatment. "I kept my mind busy making crafts or food to take my mind off chemo," Pati said. "At Christmastime we had the 'Twelve Days of Chemo' and I made something different every day for the staff members," she adds with a hearty laugh.

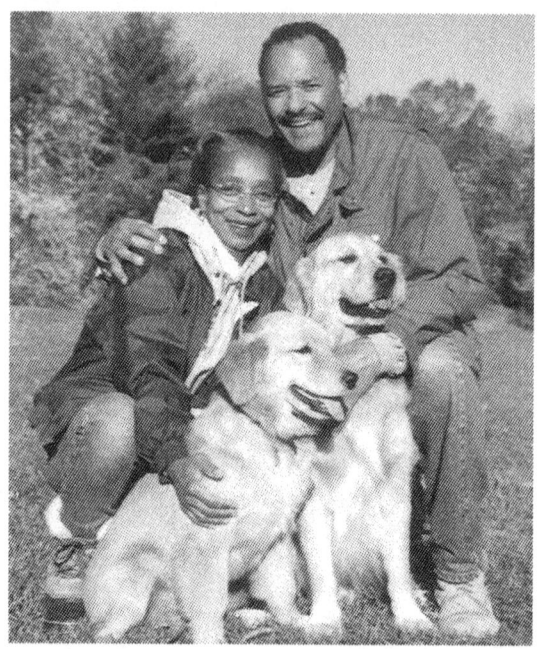

Frank A. Bolden, 58

Married 37 years, with sons 35 and 32, and a niece and nephew 26 and 24 "we call them our daughter and son" and a granddaughter.

Frank is a Vice President at Johnson & Johnson, responsible for all employee services at the headquarter offices in New Brunswick, NJ. He has a staff of about 100. Part of his background includes his 12 years as a lawyer for J&J.

Born: Albany, GA. Live: Berkley Heights, NJ.

Tumor Type: Prostate Cancer diagnosed 1998.

Treatment: Prostate was removed by surgery.

Frank supports the *National Medical Fellowship* at 5 Hanover Square, 15th floor, NY, NY 10004. They are dedicated to increasing the number of minority physicians and can be found on the web at www.nmfonline.org

Photo Credit: Sara Gold.

THERE IS A TOMORROW

"I no longer have bladder spasms nor do I need Viagra," is the good news reported by Frank Bolden, a 58-year-old prostate cancer survivor.

A lawyer and Fortune 500 corporate executive, Frank also reports that he has learned to refocus his priorities, realizing that he is not as indispensable at work as he originally envisioned. While he failed to realize this after his serious bout with diverticulitis years before, he finally learned the lesson after his cancer diagnosis.

"My leave of absence was right in the midst of a major project, and my staff went through it with flying colors without my help," Frank laughs. "It was an eye opener because I always thought that I had to be at work seven days a week to get things done. The experience changed the way I look at things."

The lessons didn't always come easily, as Frank embarked on his cancer experience with a big dose of denial. "My doctor had a sense that something might be wrong when PSA levels began to fluctuate quite a bit," Frank remembers. His primary care physician became concerned after one of his physicals and encouraged him to see a urologist. "For six months I walked around with the information in my wallet, until a colleague of mine died of colon cancer. That's when I set up the appointment." Not long after, a biopsy confirmed cancer.

Frank underwent successful surgery, and the whole experience was life changing. "I was always go, go, go," he reports, "a Type A personality who really believed that my family came first. It's now clear to me why a stronger argument could be made that my career was number one, with my family finishing a not-so-close second."

Throughout the process, Frank conducted research on the internet, participated in support groups, and relied heavily on his faith, his wife and his friends. Now cancer-free, he has learned to cultivate a life outside of work, which he has found to be extremely rewarding.

"I play tennis quite a bit, read a lot, go the theater and am active on a number of charitable and community boards," he reports. "Out of an interest in tracing my roots, I have become involved in geneology, and I've traced my great grandfather back to a plantation in New Charleston." Now close to retirement, he has set his sights on writing poetry and possibly a play.

Frank also supports other prostate cancer patients in understanding that the "c" word doesn't have to mean the end. "Don't ever think you have to go through this alone; this is a good time to begin learning that you can rely on other people," he advises.

Another piece of advice he gives people—which he admits is most readily ignored—is not to rush back to work. "If they got along without you for 6 weeks, they can get along without you for 7," Frank quips.

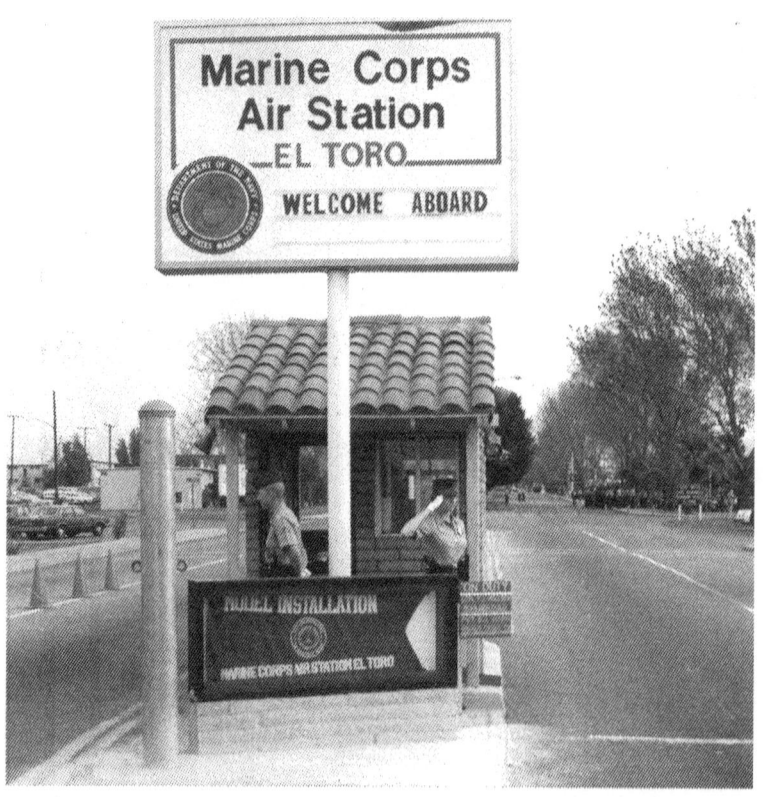

Ericka Hedlin, 35

Separated, with son Josef 10 and daughter TeiJai 15.
Ericka is an Office/Sales Manager for a publishing firm, doing database work for marketing and mailings. "And whatever I'm told to do."
Born: Martinez, California. Live: Royersford, PA
Tumor Type: Ovarian cancer (class 4) diagnosed 1985.
Treatment: One quarter of the right ovary removed, followed by radiation.
Photo Credit: Unknown.

MARINES IMPROVISE, ADAPT AND OVERCOME

You wouldn't think that too many life experiences could compare with the intensity of living alone since fifteen years of age, being a female Black Belt and serving in the U.S. Marine Corps Military Police. Think again.

"I met my boyfriend in the Marine Corps," recalls Erika Hedlin, 35-year-old ovarian cancer survivor. "My menstrual cycles were irregular, which we attributed to the rigorous physical training of the Marines. Further medical testing revealed two incredible findings—I had ovarian cancer *and* I was three months pregnant."

Erika opted to forgo treatment for cancer until her daughter was born, expecting this to be her only child. Her radiation began just a week following the birth of daughter TJ, now 13.

"I went back to work in less than three weeks and married my boyfriend shortly after," Erika explained. Within a very short time, she suffered another personal tragedy: her husband's infidelity.

"When my daughter was only six weeks old, I thought I was tough—running six miles a day, standing duty, going out in the field for weeks at a time. When I learned of his cheating, I was heartbroken—once again I thought I would die."

Through her experiences with cancer and a failed marriage, she held close to family beliefs, despite growing up amid alcoholism and sexual abuse. "My great grandmother was Native American and raised on a reservation. She was a tough cookie—she could outride any cowboy I ever knew. But she also had such grace and majesty and forgiveness."

"She taught me that even in your heart, if you think you're making a right choice, you could be making the wrong one if you're blinded by other factors—love, hurt or just plain stupidity—but that doesn't mean you can't make good choices later on. Most of all, she taught me that if you can respect yourself, then you can love yourself."

Erika pulled together and life went on, through annual medical exams and clean bills of health. Until just over a year ago...

"My doctor found a lump in my breast and I underwent a biopsy," Erika explained. "For five tortuous days, I had no idea what was in store for me. Finally, I was told it was a benign mass."

Throughout her experiences—good and bad—cancer has been a powerful teacher. "I've learned two lessons," Erika said. "As afraid as you are, there is someone out there who's had it worse and survived. And no matter what you believe in, you're never alone. In my case, God's been looking out for me big time!"

"Cancer motivated the hell out of me, because if cancer's going to catch my butt it's going to have a long run. If you let it get you down, it will get you down."

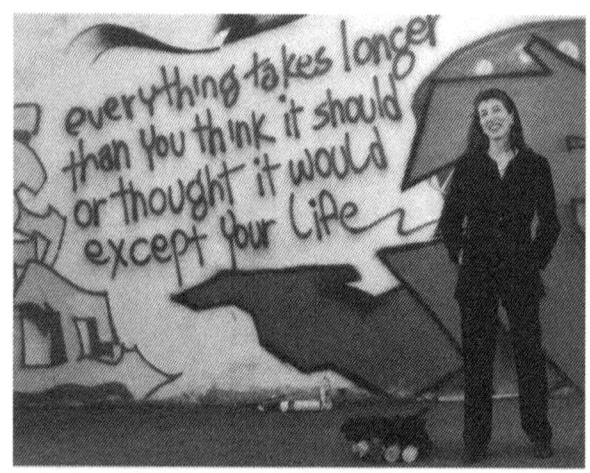

Merijane Block, 48 "And Proud of it".

Living with her partner Paul of 12 years.

*Merijane is the program manager for **The Breast Cancer Fund**, on the web at www.breastcancerfund.org, a San Francisco-based, national non-profit organization that's dedicated to identifying and eliminating the preventable causes of breast cancer, particularly those in the environment. She oversees conference, educational and advocacy programs, and coordinates "Art.Rage.Us, The Art and Outrage of Breast Cancer", an exhibit of art and writing by women with breast cancer.*

Born: Brooklyn, New York. Live: San Francisco, CA.

Tumor Type: Metastatic Breast Cancer first diagnosed April 1991.

Treatment: Lumpectomy April 15, 1992, followed by radiation in June and July. Local recurrence in November 1994, followed by mastectomy January 31, 1995. Radiation treatment in Fall of 1996 for metastasis to the spine, which recurred in 1999. Ongoing treatment with Aredia (a bone-building drug) and Tamoxifen. "I've also been working with a nice Jewish boy who is a wonderful Chinese Medicine practitioner."

Photo Credit: Friend, fellow breast cancer survivor and Art.Rage.Us. artist, Nancy Bellen.

FEARLESS SELF EXPRESSION

Forty-eight-year-old breast cancer fighter (she doesn't call herself a survivor) Merijane Block says that realism in addressing cancer as a chronic disease, not as a "lesson" you need to learn, has helped her survive—and thrive—for the past decade.

"Growing up, cancer was this big secret nobody ever talked about," she said. "And, God forbid you had breast cancer—having a breast cut off meant that you were no longer a woman."

Merijane approached her diagnosis of breast cancer head-on, finding and using the words "fearless self-expression" as her guide.

"I just felt that if I could always make the effort to fearlessly express myself, then I would be able to save myself," she remarked. "I use the word 'save' knowing that it is very different from 'cure.' Now, I see myself as a healthy person living with cancer."

Throughout her therapy, writing was her primary form of fearless self-expression. Some of that writing, including the poem that is shown in graffiti in her photo, appears in the book "Art.Rage.Us, Art and Writing by Women with Breast Cancer", the companion book to the exhibit, which has received nationwide recognition.

"My triumph is my work in the world," says Merijane. "I have the ability to demystify cancer for people by speaking about it very matter-of-factly. I want people to get over the notion that cancer has to be a secret or that breast cancer has to be shameful."

Her personal commitment to demystifying breast cancer is evidenced by the fact that she doesn't wear a prosthesis. "I make it a point not to hide that I have one breast. Maybe the biggest triumph of my life is to make women understand that they are whole no matter what," Merijane said.

Unlike other people with cancer, "I don't think it's made my life better, but my response to the challenges of cancer has made my life better," she explained. "I don't believe that cancer is a gift or a lesson you have to learn, but that we're ordinary people in an extraordinary situation. While we can't always control the cancer, we can control our response to it. In fact, it may be the only control we have."

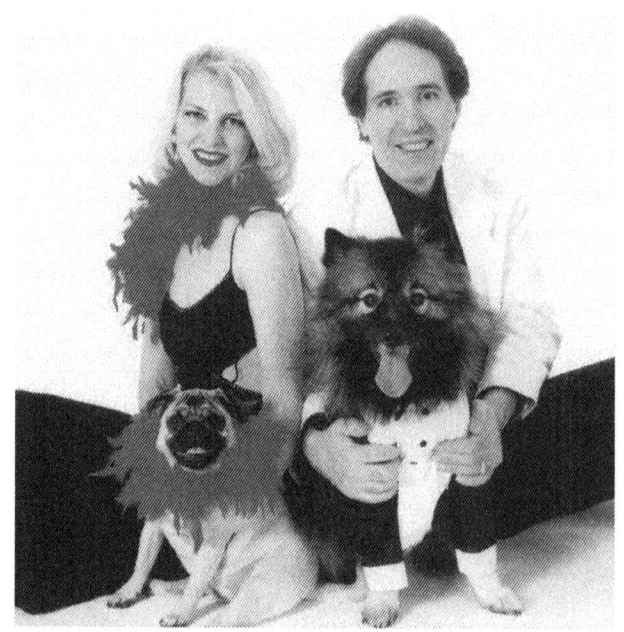

Edward Leigh, 42

Married 7 years to Beth, no children. "Five dogs and four cats are our kids."
*Eddie is a motivational speaker and seminar leader who helps people find joy
in the workplace and classroom. "How to make things more fun, interesting
and creative."*
Born: Cleveland, OH. Lives: Cleveland, OH
Tumor Type: Colon cancer diagnosed August 1999.
Treatment: Chemotherapy plus removal of ascending colon, part of the
small intestine, appendix and local lymph nodes.
Eddie supports the Colon Cancer Alliance. He can be reached through his
company, Edward Leigh Enterprises at 800-677-3256 and by his website
www.EdwardLeigh.com.
Photo Credit: MotoPhoto.

SEMICOLON SAYS 'CHECK YOUR ASS FOR A MASS'

He keeps his surgical staples in a glass jar, believing that it's better to crack up from laughter than from stress.

Edward Leigh is a motivational speaker who was diagnosed with colon cancer in 1999, after two years of misdiagnoses by another doctor.

He had surgery—wearing a clown's nose—to remove his ascending colon, a portion of his small intestine, his appendix and all of the lymph nodes in the surrounding area. After surgery, he realized it was painful to laugh. But within a few weeks, he was back to laughing on a regular basis. Eddie believes that it's better to crack up from laughter than from stress.

He experienced severe nausea and vomiting from the ten months of chemotherapy that followed and lost some of his hair. "The worst part of my treatment was when I came home and I'd see Joan Rivers on Larry King and I always got a kick out of her—I started laughing and then suddenly I realized that after abdominal surgery, laughter can be a painful thing."

Eddie found people incredibly compassionate during his recovery. "I thought my clients would write me off," Eddie remarked. "But, to my surprise, they were wonderful," Eddie reports. "They rescheduled events to accommodate my treatment schedule, and sent me flowers and fruit baskets every month."

According to Eddie, many people think he became a motivational speaker after his cancer diagnosis, but it was actually before. "I may have gotten more business since I've gotten cancer, but I do tell other speakers I do not recommend getting cancer as a marketing tool," he says with a laugh.

Strangers also reached out to Eddie during his treatment. When he ordered pizza, cake and flowers for his health care team upon finishing chemo, "I remember picking up the flowers at the local florist, when the florist saw the cake and asked me what it was for," he said. "She was so touched that she started to cry. She told me to pick out a balloon, attached some candy to it. I asked her how much, and she said, 'just a thank you. This is my gift.'"

Even his pets stayed by his side. "When I was in chemo, one day I threw up and it was so rough that there were tears in my eyes," Eddie recounts. "Molly, one of our dogs, jumped on the bed and came up to my face and she licked the tears out of my eye. It was almost like it was her way of trying to make me feel better."

Another highlight of his treatment—he has many positive memories—was joining a colon cancer online discussion group and finding out that the survivors called themselves "semicolons." "I even had a little button made up with the punctuation mark on it," Eddie said. "I walk around with the button and explain to people what it actually means. A friend of mine suggested that I tell people I'm half-assed, but I like the term 'semicolon' a little better."

A few years later, Eddie's now just a happy, healthy person "who happened to develop cancer," a term he learned from a close friend and cancer survivor. "I don't like to use the term 'cancer patient' because the word 'cancer' comes first. I think I'm a person first," he remarked.

Eddie the wisecracker does have a few wise words for others. "One of the most important messages I can leave people, as sick as it sounds, is to 'check your ass for a mass.' It may sound offensive, but if you remember to do it, then I've done my job."

With cancer behind him, so to speak, life is good. "As long as I wake up in the morning and I'm breathing I know it's going to be a good day," he expressed.

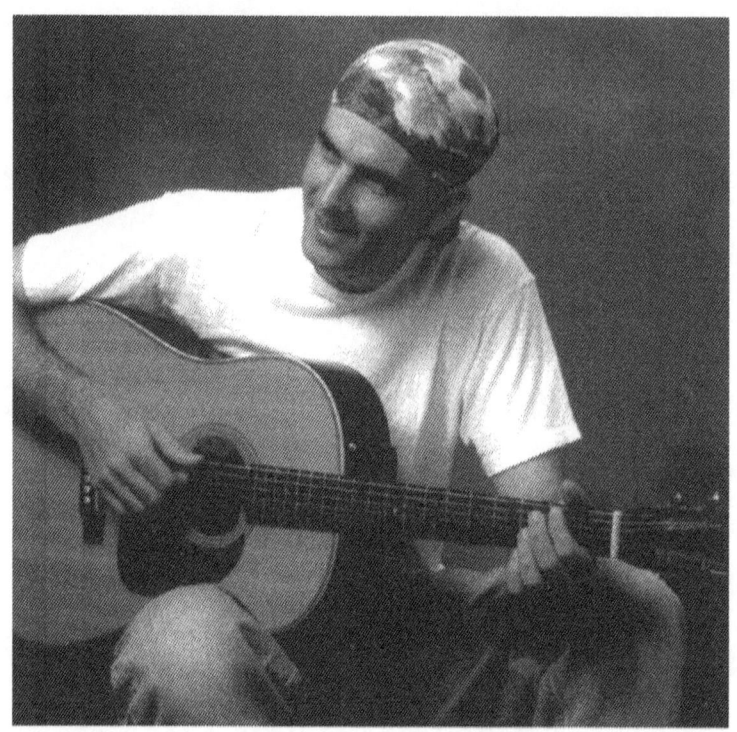

David M. Bailey, 35

Married 12 years to Leslie, with daughter Kelcey (9) and son Cameron (7). *David is a performing songwriter, and has performed in 36 states and at many cancer benefit concerts. David's five albums, "Peace," "Love the Time," "One More Day," "Life," and a live album are all available at his website, davidmbailey.com. His sixth album, "Grace", will be released Fall of 2001.* Born: Pittsburgh, PA. Lives: Stafford, VA
Tumor Type: GBM Brain Cancer diagnosed June, 1996.
Treatment: 2 surgeries, 4 different chemos and radiation.
David supports the American Brain Tumor Association, the National Brain Tumor Foundation in San Francisco, and the Brain Tumor Society in Boston and adds, "I love Duke University."
Photo Credit—Unknown

ONE MORE DAY

When you're diagnosed with cancer, every day that you get to start over is the dawn of a new statistic.

In the words of David Bailey, a 35-year-old brain cancer survivor, statistics regarding your prognosis are required in the medical community, but have little merit for those actually fighting the disease.

"Statistics are what doctors and scientists use to discuss the universe of patients, not what survivors should use," David explained. "Every day, you get to start over and begin a new statistic. I think doctors should say 'these are numbers, but there are lots and lots of people who break them and you can be a statistical anomaly, too.'"

David's cancer was diagnosed in an emergency situation after he experienced severe headaches. "Four days after getting into an ambulance following extreme nausea, I woke up in an emergency room in a hospital about 50 miles from my home. The doctors reported that I had a brain tumor the size of a baseball," he remembers.

He emerged from surgery alive, but with mixed reviews. While surgeons successfully removed the tumor, David's cancer had already progressed to stage four, which carried with it a statistical survival of less than one year.

"I went to an oncologist and asked if a situation like mine is always lethal," David remarked. "The doctor shrugged his shoulders and told me that what I had was hard to beat."

Unwilling to accept that his life was approaching the end, David conducted extensive research on the internet and found a new oncologist at Duke University, a major cancer institution. "Dr. Friedman TOLD me to come down and page him, and that he would see me immediately. He said, 'I understand you have a brain tumor. This is what we're going to do about it.' It was great to believe in a doctor and to stop worrying as much, knowing that he would take care of me." David arrived late at night and paged the doctor from the lobby of the hospital. The doctor came right away.

David's conversations with his doctors were followed by intense dialogue with God. "I imagined a conversation with God and I wondered what would happen if I asked every question and He answered them. Then I thought, the better question isn't 'why', but 'what now?' and that was the last time I asked why."

David's cancer experience also helped to patch "a hole in his heart," nonsurgically speaking. "About a week after the first surgery I was sitting out in the back yard. I had given up playing the guitar while I was in the working world. In retrospect, it left a huge hole in my heart. My wife, Leslie, walked out back and gave me my guitar without saying anything. I began to cry because I didn't know if I'd be able to play again."

He was able to play, and this moment launched his professional music career. David has since recorded five albums and performed in 35 states, often at cancer benefit concerts. His fifth album will be released soon.

"Through my music, I have been able to reach out to others with my gifts," David remarked. "When I perform, I pass my thoughts and insights to the audience and urge them to find their dreams, pursue their passion and appreciate the moment. It's a constant reminder to myself that I can never again allow myself or the people around me to take a single day for granted, nor accept anything less than what our pure passion is."

For David, each day now represents a new beginning. "In the song that I perform at the end of my concerts, 'One More Day,' I say that if you wake up with another day, say 'hallelujah' that your time here isn't done yet, and realize that God is voting 'yes' to giving you another chance to do something really important with your life."

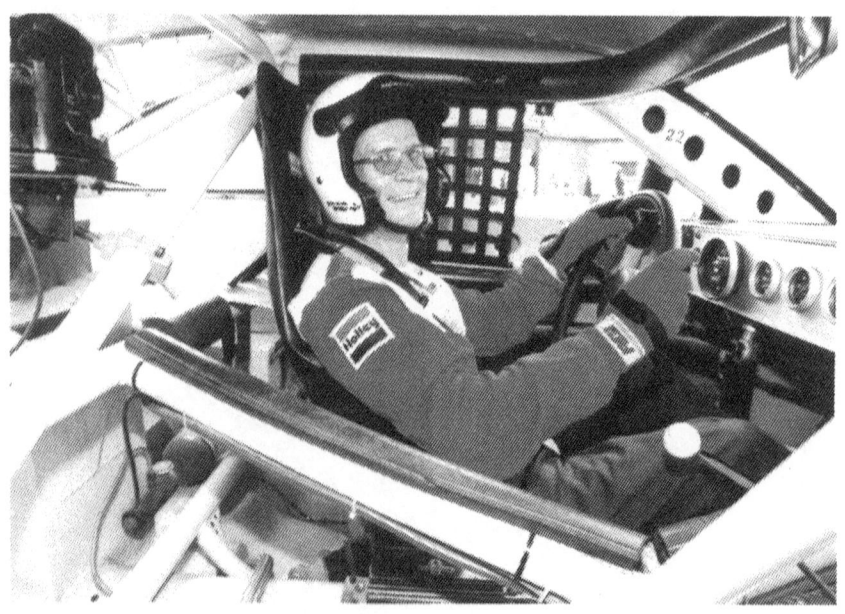

John R. Conway, 62

Married 16 years (second marriage), with children and stepchildren from 28 to 40, plus 12 grandchildren.

John sold power equipment for 35 years before retiring January 2001.

Born: Carrollton, GA. Live: Thoroughfair, NJ.

Tumor Type: Esophageal diagnosed July 1998.

Treatment: Chemotherapy and radiation followed by removal of the esophagus. John supports various children's cancer charities.

Photo Credit: Unknown. John in Dover, Delaware at day of racing.

GENTLEMEN, START YOUR ENGINES!

He wasn't going to die because he wasn't ready and his wife wouldn't let him.

John Conway, esophageal cancer survivor, credits his great family, great doctors and unwillingness to die as the cornerstones in his battle to survive.

"My family helped a lot. I would never have made it without my wife—she was positive, saying, 'You're not going to leave me here by myself. You're not dying because you're not allowed!'"

Years ago, John underwent surgery for gastric reflux and a hiatle hernia, but two years ago, he began to experience heartburn that he hadn't had before. An esophageal tumor was discovered during endoscopy and he immediately underwent chemotherapy, radiation and, six weeks later, surgery.

He has tremendous confidence in his medical team, a father-son duo at Thomas Jefferson Medical Center in Philadelphia. "In simplified terms, the surgeons removed my esophagus and then stretched my stomach up to meet the other end," John said. Every three months since, he has an outpatient procedure in which a balloon catheter is inserted in order to "stretch" his throat. One of the procedures resulted in a life-threatening infection. He has also weathered the administration of some experimental treatments because of his unique cancer type. "My medical file is about four inches thick," John remarked.

Despite surgery and stretches, he feels that he is one of the "lucky ones." "I didn't lose my hair during chemotherapy and I didn't get sick until the last week, which was still relatively minor. I was on prayer lists all over the country, and I know that had a lot to do with how good I felt."

John's medical team—his surgeon, family physician, oncologist and radiation oncologist—all credit his recovery in great part to his positive attitude and sense of humor.

When he received phone calls from well-wishers, they were clearly concerned about his ability to survive. "I'd tell all of them, 'I not dying. I'm going to beat this thing because I'm going to see all of my grandkids get married."

He added, "Now that I'm still living, people have told me that they believe there was a purpose to my cancer. I don't know if I fully understand that concept yet, but I am certainly more aware of my health and I take better care of myself than I did before my diagnosis."

John and his wife now take walks in the park and fish from their boat— activities he expects to do more of as his strength continues to improve. He also has begun to give back as a result of his cancer experience, serving as a "phone buddy" for newly diagnosed patients at Thomas Jefferson. Following his retirement, he also plans to spend time working with children who have cancer.

John's advice for the newly diagnosed: be positive, involve your family and find a medical team you can trust. "If you find out you have cancer, accept it and fight like heck because you're the only one who's going to control it. You're going to get more support from your family than you are from anybody else. Your doctors can do amazing things, but if you don't have a positive attitude and if you don't let your family and friends help, then you're not doing all you can to beat it," John said.

Now and into the future, John has every intention of living life to the fullest. "For Christmas, my wife gave me a day in Dover, Delaware, where I got to drive a race car around the track. I have the plaque and picture to prove it. Here I am a cancer survivor at almost 62 years old driving a racecar at 130 miles per hour. How great is that?!"

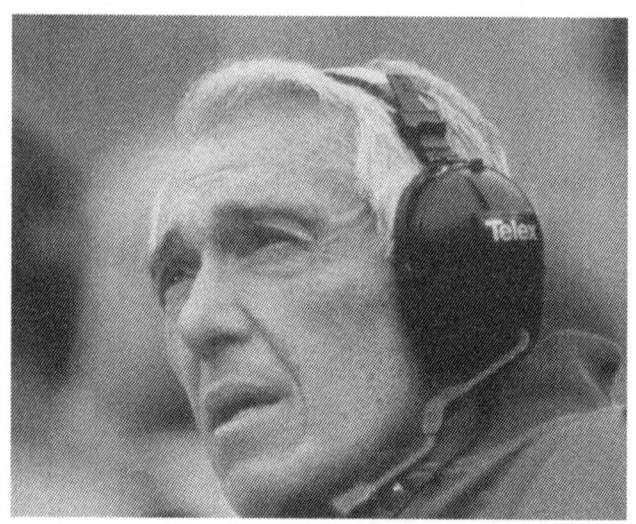

Marv Levy, 75

Married 7 years (second marriage) with one daughter (32).
Marv is a retired NFL football coach (Buffalo Bills) and led his team to four Super Bowl appearances in his total of 47 years coaching. He now works as an analyst for the Fox sports cable network show "NFL This Morning" every Sunday.
Born: Chicago, IL. Lives: Chicago, IL
Tumor Type: Prostate cancer diagnosed July 1995.
Treatment: Surgical removal of the prostate.
Photo Credit: Buffalo Bills.

WHEN THE GENERAL TELLS ME TO MARCH I MARCH

In cancer, as in football, records are made to be broken.

"When I asked my doctor how long I'd be out after my surgery, he said that the average was six to eight weeks and his record was four weeks. "I was back coaching in three weeks," remarks Marv Levy, retired Buffalo Bills football coach.

Upon receiving his biopsy results after having elevated PSA levels for two consecutive years, Levy said he was in disbelief that he had prostate cancer. "I sought three more opinions and they verified the original results," he said. "I didn't know where to turn."

Once he got his bearings, he called everyone he knew who had prostate cancer, including Len Dawson, former quarterback with the Kansas City Chiefs, and a coach on his Bills staff. "Once you're over the shock, it's important to begin to assemble all the information you can and take things one step at a time, rather than just lying in a fetal position," he advises.

After conducting research, Marv considered waiting until the end of the season to seek treatment, but the Bills team owner Ralph Wilson convinced him otherwise. "He grabbed me by the shirt, shook his head and said, 'Oh, no, no. You won't wait until the end of the season. You go now and don't worry about us.'"

At the age of 70, Marv opted for an aggressive approach to treatment—surgery to remove his prostate—and banked blood in preparation for the procedure. He admits to having been in very good shape for his age, running three miles a day and lifting weights.

"You don't know until you wake up from surgery how accurate the doctors' original characterizations of the cancer are," he remarked.

"Luckily, the surgeons said my cancer was confined, my prostate was removed and I had a strong likelihood of being cured."

During his three-week recovery, Marv received a call from General Schwartzkopf, U.S. troop commander during the Gulf War and fellow prostate cancer survivor, who told him to start walking as soon as he could. "If the general tells me to march, I'm going to march," Marv jokes. "And I'm still marching to this day."

After cancer, Marv says he more readily appreciates the simple things in life, like the change of seasons. "When I walked back into the stadium, I realized how fortunate I was to walk down that tunnel, and I never appreciated my friends or family more," he remembers. "I was truly thankful for the gift of life."

Marv adds, "Like football, I can say that cancer doesn't build character, it reveals character."

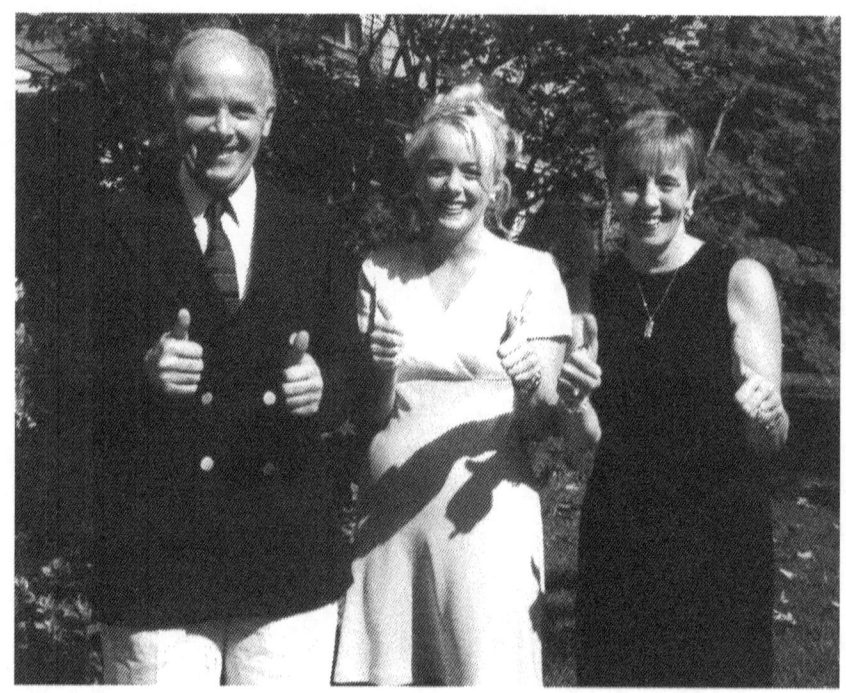

Christina Smillie, 25

Single
Christina is a product specialist for Ortho Biotech and sells oncology drugs.
Born: Youngstown Ohio. Lives: Carmel, IN
Tumor Type: Paraganglioma (a parasympathetic nervous system tumor) diagnosed March 1991, with main tumor in stomach. Metastases to the brain, kidney and thigh.
Treatment: Radioactive drug given intravenously.
Photo Credit: Christina's sister Fiona Smillie.

I HAVE CANCER, BUT CANCER DOESN'T HAVE ME

"I had more life experience before I was 16 than some people have in a lifetime."

The words of cancer survivor Christina Smillie refer to open heart surgery as a young child, followed by her father's testicular cancer and her own diagnosis of Paraganglioma.

"I was 16, and on the homecoming court and a cheerleader," she remembers. I kept thinking 'This doesn't happen to people like me.' I couldn't believe I was going to get my head cut open."

Christina's cancer was discovered after she experienced terrific stomach pain nearly all of the time; she was also suffering the emotional effects caused from the tumor's release of hormones in her body.

At her insistence, her gynecologist reluctantly proceeded with an ultrasound, which diagnosed her tumor. The surgery to have it removed was performed on April Fool's Day. Following considerable research on the part of her mother, who is a nurse, Christina then entered an experimental treatment protocol. She needed to travel to her therapy by plane as a participant in the "Angel Flights" program, a charity that donates unused corporate jet time to cancer patients.

Her protocol included high doses of a radioactive drug given intravenously. "I wasn't expected to do well," Christina recalls. "I was sicker than anything. I couldn't eat, drink or chew and couldn't swallow because my mouth was so dry." She also experienced pain and debilitating fatigue, which necessitated repeated blood transfusions, from which she was infected with hepatitis C. "People would tell me how brave I was. What choice did I have?" Christina remarked.

Now 25, Christina is a pharmaceutical sales representative, and has built her first house. In her professional role of selling treatments for cancer patients, she once again is no stranger to infusion centers.

"I can honestly tell patients that I know what they're going through," Christina reports. "It's easy to bond with them because of our mutual experience, and I give them hope by telling them how long I've been tumor-free. Through my job, I feel like I'm making a difference and touching people's lives."

Stemming from her experiences and her love of children, Christina has also served as a mentor at a treatment center for children who have been taken into state's custody. "Giving anyone hope isn't false hope, because I wasn't supposed to make it and here I am. Even with a small chance, there's still a chance," she says. "Fighting, treatment and attitude equal success in a lot of cases."

"I heard a quote once: 'I have cancer, but cancer doesn't have me.' I truly believe that."

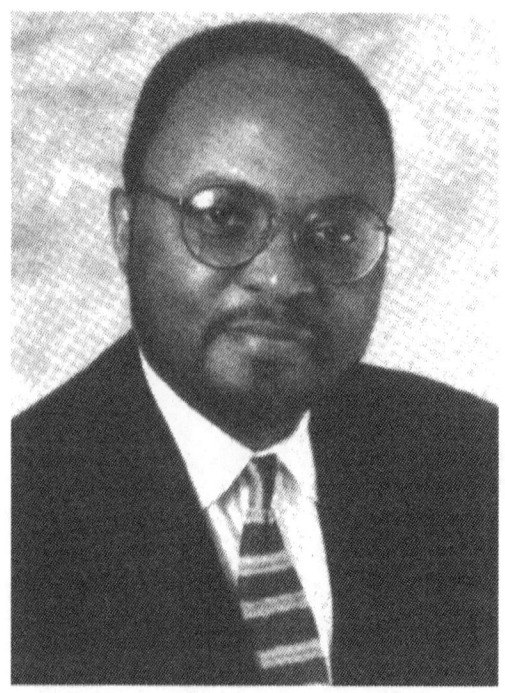

Ed Hill, 48

Married 5 years to Brenda (second marriage), with two sons and two daughters 19 to 25.

Ed is the Vice President of Human Resources for Janssen Pharmaceutica a division of Johnson and Johnson

Born: Gary, Indiana. Live: Newtown, PA

Tumor Type: Multiple Myeloma diagnosed in the Fall of 1998.

Treatment: An allogeneic (from another person) bone marrow transplant along with chemotherapy.

Ed supports, among other charities, the Multiple Myeloma Research Foundation and is now friends with its director, Kathy Giusti (see her interview).

Photo Credit: Cancer Care.

GRACE UNDER PRESSURE

Being independent his entire life, this corporate executive found it difficult to place the call to tell his siblings about his cancer, much less about his need for a bone marrow donor.

"I finally decided to let the whole family know and have them tested to see if there would be a match for an allogeneic bone marrow transplant," Ed said. "Those were difficult calls to make—calling your sisters and your brothers to say, 'I have cancer and I need your help.'"

Ed's diagnosis came when his annual physical detected a blood chemistry abnormality. Further tests confirmed Multiple Myeloma. "I thought that everything I'd worked for and everything I'd become was going down the tubes," Ed remembers.

His doctors told him that he needed to act quickly, and his family rallied around him with a unanimous response to help in any way they could. "They all went for the bone marrow blood test and my little sister Denise, who is five years younger than me, turned out to be the bone marrow match that ended up saving my life," Ed remarked.

"She volunteered to go through the pain of the bone marrow harvest process in order give me a second chance at life," he continued. "And this was a woman with nine children between the ages of eight and 29 who had already made a lot of sacrifices in her life for the sake of others," he added. "I let her know every day how indebted I am to her and that I love her for caring enough to help me beat this disease."

Despite some serious side effects along the way, including the inability to walk for three weeks, Ed's cancer is now in full remission, and his bone marrow has been almost totally replaced by his sister's transplanted marrow.

The experience has strengthened his relationship with his wife and siblings, and also with his extended family. "I have started to actively reach out beyond my immediate brothers and sisters to include my nieces and nephews and my cousins," Ed said. "If you don't believe me, look at how my telephone bill has tripled in the past 12 months." Ed has also supported others who are newly diagnosed, including friends at work and their families.

Now in remission, Ed and Brenda have moved to a new house in the country, the construction of which she supervised during his treatment. "I was very blessed that the good Lord above had given me a woman who could be by my side and help me through the whole process."

For him, every day is a gift. "Life is too precious—remember that tomorrow's not promised to anyone," he said. "Moreover, in the midst of your cancer experience, realize that this too shall pass. Remember that there are people who will help you along the way, and do the same for others."

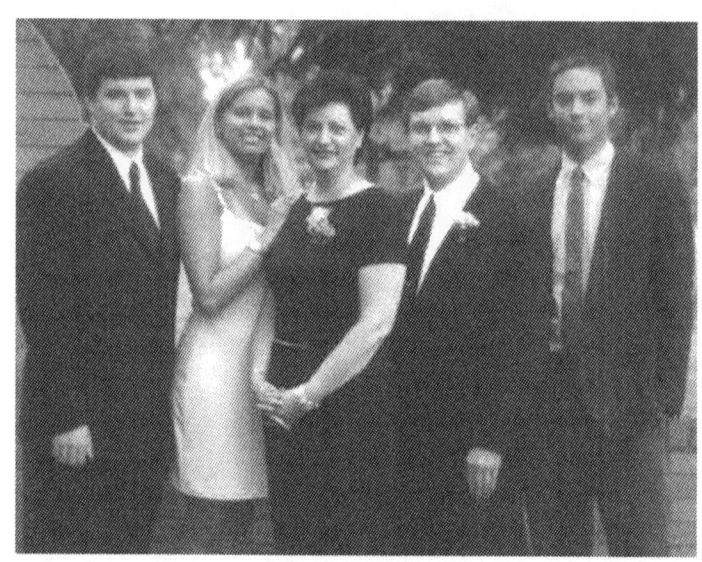

Michael H. Miller, 49

Son Michael (24), daughter Jena (17), wife Judy, Michael, and son Chris (21). *Michael is retired after 22 years as a competitive swimming coach. He is now a prostate cancer survivor activist and works with the National Prostate Cancer Coalition. Mike also started a foundation in Juno called the "Southeast Alaska Cancer and Wellness Foundation," whose mission is to empower people by bringing health and wellness resources together. Also, Mike was selected to be a TorchBearer prior to the 2002 Winter Olympic Games, and will carry the torch in Juneau, Alaska on January 24, 2002.*
Born: Portland, OR. Lives: Juno, AK (for 19 years), returning to Portland, OR.
Tumor Type: Metastatic Prostate Cancer (stage D2), diagnosed January 17, 1996, with one recurrence.
Treatment: A clinical trial program of various chemotherapeutic and hormonal agents.
Photo Credit: Unknown Family Member.

THE RIGHT SIDE OF THE PLANE

His son is his hero.

Michael Miller is the survivor of two family crises—his son's near-fatal accident and his own prostate cancer.

"My oldest son was hit by a truck and given only a 2 percent chance of living," Mike explained. "Now 24, he's the guy who taught me how to face my cancer—he's my hero. I spent six of the seven months with him during his recovery."

Mike's diagnosis was made after the typical symptom of difficulty in urinating. "The doctor told me that I had a metastatic cancer that was aggressive and had spread to the bones," Mike recalls. "I was given three years to live." Mike noted that his physician urged him to seek a second opinion, which he did, and it confirmed the original diagnosis.

Mike entered a clinical trial of various chemotherapeutic and hormonal agents. His PSA levels went from a high of 26.6 to a low of zero in just six weeks, the tumors on his skull and vertebrae were totally eradicated and he is now considered stable. However, he did experience significant side effects from the treatments, including hearing loss, and he still needs to take various hormonal supplements.

Mike has been active in support groups, and has taken several incidents as signs that the angels were on his side from the start. "When we flew down to Oregon for my second opinion, I was on the right hand side of the plane where it was sunny," he remembers. "The left hand side was cloudy—it was like there was a dividing line. Every time I focused on the right hand side of the plane I had a great deal of energy. I decided then that I was going to stay on the right side of the plane, which is where I've been ever since."

At times Mike was so afraid of dying that he saw angels in his dreams.

"When I attended my first support group, I opened the door to pitch blackness, and saw the participants passing a candle to commemorate a woman who died of breast cancer," he remembers. "The way they talked about her death and how she lived her life alleviated any fears I had of dying. I could finally face my own mortality head on instead of living in constant fear."

After his cancer experience, Mike has spoken to schools and the community regularly, in his home state of Alaska, throughout the western United States, and in Washington, D.C., before Congress and the Defense Department.

Much of his work has been directed toward increasing government funding and insurance coverage for prostate cancer diagnosis and treatment. Mike was instrumental in getting Alaska to require insurance carriers to pay for PSA tests for high-risk men (African American or those with a family history) at age 35 instead of 40, and for everyone age 40 instead of 50. He has been honored with awards from the state of Alaska in recognition of his work.

Mike feels that his work stems from responsibility and the ability to respond. "I had the will to live and the mental toughness it takes," Mike reflects. "As a survivor, I want to respond in kind to the community that gave me so much when I needed its help."

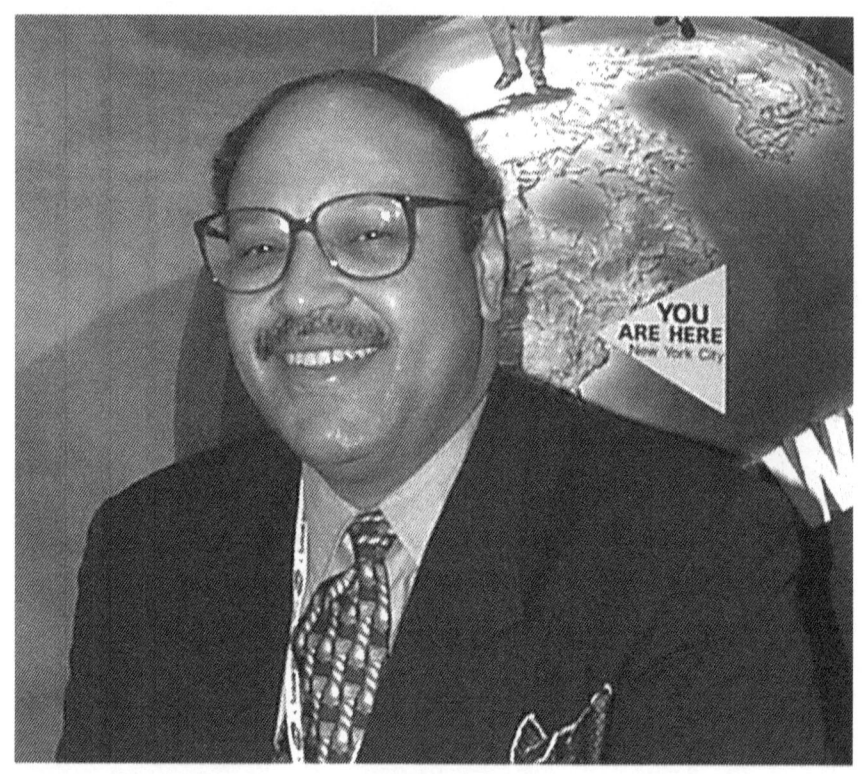

Virgil H. Simons, 55

Married to Jennifer for 30 years.

Virgil is General Manager of Dogi USA, Inc., a fabric manufacturer.

Born: Chicago, IL. Lives: Secaucus, NJ.

Tumor Type: Prostate Cancer diagnosed April 1995.

Treatment: Radical prostatectomy.

Virgil established a non-profit foundation to help others fight the disease, and can be reached at "The Prostate Net", P.O. Box 2192, Secaucus, NJ 07096, or online at www.prostate-online.com

Photo Credit: Unknown.

PATHS TO EMPOWERMENT

"I stopped wearing watches," remarked Virgil Simons, a 55-year-old prostate cancer survivor. "Watches make you think about the time you need to spend in the future, rather than the time you are living now."

Following a diagnosis of prostate cancer, Virgil underwent a radical prostatectomy. "When you have cancer, you can't surrender your life to anyone," he said. "I decided that this was my life, and I was going to live it on my own terms regardless of the outcome. I knew that I had way too much ahead of me to give up."

After successful surgery, Virgil channeled his energy and conviction into establishing a non-profit foundation to help others fight the disease. Remarkably, he now says, "Getting cancer was the best thing that could have happened to me. It helped me to look beyond superficial things that I once viewed as important to realizing what really matters in my life."

His cancer experience has enabled him to form life-long friendships with other prostate cancer survivors, including Manny Vazquez (see his interview). "Manny was one of those unseen voices on the Internet who gave me insights and encouragement," Virgil explained. "His support empowered me to make the decisions that ultimately saved my life."

And what a fine life it is, according to Virgil. "Anything can make me smile—the sun peering through a cloudy sky, playing with my dog, hitting a great backhand on the tennis court," he reports. "I'm now able to find the pleasures that exist everyday."

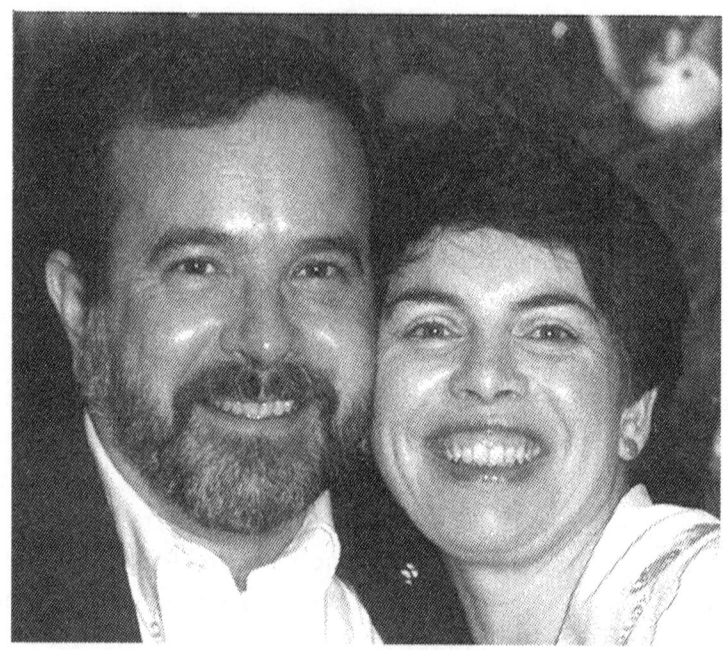

Manuel Vazquez, 61

Married (second marriage) for 16 years to Mary, with four boys age 38, 35, 34 and 31, and two girls, ages 36 and 29.

Manny is retired from 30 years in the Texaco Information Services Division, working in Network and Computer Operations.

Born: Havana, Cuba. Lives: Houston, TX. (Since 1962)

Tumor Type: Adenocarcinoma with three diploid tumors confined to the prostate gland, diagnosed 1994.

Treatment: Radical prostatectomy.

Manny is involved in countless charities, among them "TEX-US TOO Prostate Cancer Support Group." He also contributed to the book "Prostate Cancer: Portraits of Empowerment" now on sale at major bookstores. He has been invited to speak in Barcelona, Spain.

Photo Credit: Don Andrews

A VERY SIMPLE, ORDINARY HUMAN BEING

Manuel Vasquez knows adversity all too well.

Upon arriving in the United States from Cuba in the early '60s, he worked for 50 cents an hour in a car wash and scraped food off garbage cans to survive.

Thirty years later, he was again fighting for his life—against prostate cancer.

"My urologist was cold, impersonal and detached," Manny said. "I was demoralized and felt desperately alone."

He reached out to a fellow employee he located through his company's human resources department, a move that had a significant impact on him.

"More than providing me with information, he served as a role model of someone who had gone through a radical prostatectomy and was still a functional, happy person," Manny said.

"However, I owe my life to my wife, who nagged me for 10 years to have a physical exam before I had one—the one that detected my cancer," Manny tells others. "Prior to my diagnosis, I paid little attention to physical exams, preventive medicine and nutrition—practices that are now a mainstay of my lifestyle. Now I am all too aware of how fragile life really is."

Following his own surgery, he channeled his anger and frustration into helping other prostate cancer patients understand that they weren't alone. Manny is active in numerous charities, including the TEX-US Too Prostate Cancer Support Group and the American Cancer Society, through which he delivers presentations on prostate cancer to civic and church groups, adult education classes and corporate wellness programs.

He is also a regular participant in Spanish-language radio programming on prostate cancer detection, and has won many awards for his work.

Manny explains his more popular talks. "I give frequent presentations to church, civic, adult education, and wellness groups on behalf of the American Cancer Society. The idea is to use familiar objects or ideas to grasp new concepts: a cucumber, lemon and grapefruit connected by drinking straws represents the male genito-urinary system. I swing the cucumber up and down while the objects are over my abdomen, and at that point I have a captive audience. Laughter invariably breaks out and people loosen up. It gets them to open up and talk."

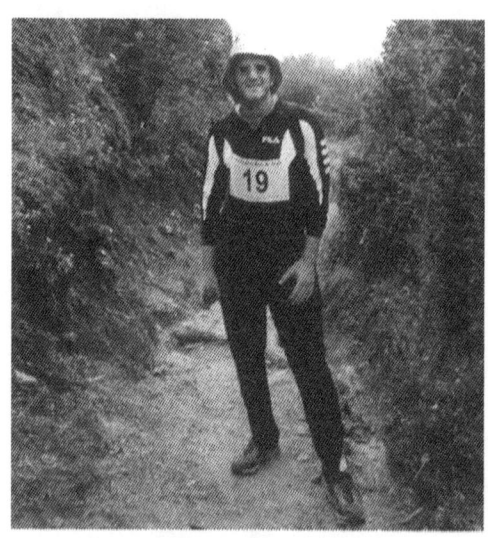

Doug Ulman, 23

Single.

Doug is the Director of Survivorship at the Lance Armstrong Foundation and previously the Executive Director of the Ulman Cancer Fund for Young Adults, a foundation that provides support resources and education to young adults, their families and friends who are affected by cancer. He remains an active board member of the fund.

Born: Columbia MD. Lives: Austin, TX.

Tumor Type: Chondrosarcoma (cartilage tumor) diagnosed August 1996, and malignant melanoma diagnosed March 1997 (on chest) and again in June 1997 (on arm).

Treatment: Surgery for all three diagnoses, rib and tumor removed for chondrosarcoma.

Doug's articles written for the Baltimore Sun on his 100-mile marathon are archived on the Fund's website, ulmanfund.org. There are many more details about the organization and its work there.

Photo Credit: Unknown. Doug on his 100 mile marathon in the Himalayan Mountains.

A LIFETIME OF OPPORTUNITY

"The tumor on my rib was discovered by a fluke after I ended up in the emergency room that August after going for a run. I was having a little problem breathing and after awhile my parents said maybe we should just go check this out. It was close to midnight so we went to the emergency room. As a young kid I had had asthma and so the doctor at the emergency room said it's probably just an allergic reaction to something. So he told me to go home and gave me an antibiotic. But as I was leaving, he said 'you know what let's just take a chest x-ray'." The next day Doug's personal physician called to tell him to get a CT scan. The tumor was lodged between his spine, lungs and ribs. "There are so many things that had to happen for him to take the chest x-ray and me to go to the hospital that I feel very fortunate it happened. I wouldn't change it for the world."

The tumor and the attached rib were removed. He didn't find out that it was cancer until the pathology reports came back. "It's a very slow growing tumor so I'm just followed now with checkups." Doug believes that his compromised immune system could have contributed to his malignant melanoma diagnoses seven and ten months later. The first was on his chest and removed. The second was invasive and removed.

"I feel great. I can't complain. I'm very active physically and do a ton of things. It's always in the back of your mind that it may come back but I feel very lucky to have had cancer at such a young age. I think that you develop an outlook on life that's very unique. Most people don't have the ability to develop that until later on."

"I think it's unique to be able to truly appreciate life. Although it sounds very cliché, when you're told you have a life threatening illness at the age of 19 you really start to understand what's important, and for me that's my family and friends."

Doug talks to his parents and brother every day now.

"I'd never been in a hospital before, so having surgery was a huge thing, only to discover that what was supposedly just a growth was cancer."

"When I was first diagnosed I was getting ready to start my sophomore year at Brown University. It's tough to be in college and go through something like this. College is just a time of hanging out with your friends and being invincible, partying, etc. To be told that you have to be different at that point because of the disease is difficult."

In 1997 he opened his foundation office in Maryland. "It's grown so fast and unfortunately there's more and more young adults out there to help. It's becoming a large population."

"When I was diagnosed, we called every 800 number and every support group and we couldn't find anything that I felt I fit into. I was referred to support groups where everybody there was over 60 and support groups for young adults and when I'd show up there wouldn't be anybody else there. It was very frustrating and I wanted to know that there were other young people out there. I was dying to find somebody who could say 'I've been there.' So I decided to start something myself.

"At first I was frustrated with a lot of people because I didn't feel like they understood what I was going through. That frustration has changed. Now I think it's because a lot of people don't know how to act around people that have cancer or get cancer or don't know how severe of a problem it is."

When asked if he's made time for hobbies, Doug quickly answers yes. "I love to run marathons now. I played soccer in college but I play more now."

Doug also mentions that he ran the one hundred mile Mount Everest Challenge Marathon in the Himalayan mountains in five days last fall. Doug ran twenty miles a day for five days with about 65 others, sleeping in cabins or tents each night. "It was quite an experience and that's something that I never would've had the opportunity to do, much less would've been interested in doing, if I hadn't had this experience."

His athletic background got his path to cross with Lance Armstrong (see his interview). "I love to tell the story of getting this email from him. It's great that somebody of his stature takes the time to send a random email."

When asked what he's learned, Doug names two things. "First I think that my mission in life is to help other people. Second is that as much as we hear the cliché that sometimes bad things have to happen to good people, there can be so many positives that come out of it. I always say when I go speak, 'The last four years of my life have been the worst by far, and they've been the best, and I wouldn't change them for anything'."

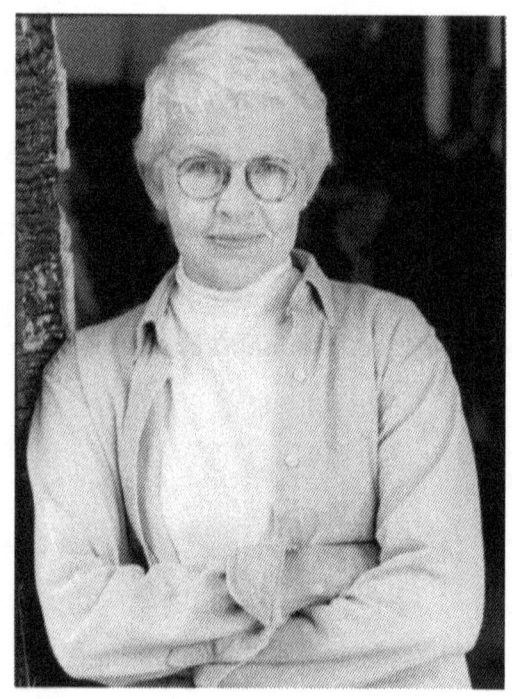

Betty DeGeneres, 70

Divorced. Betty has a son, Vance (45) and a daughter Ellen (42).
Betty is a writer and a speaker.
Born: New Orleans, LA. Live: Ojai, CA
Tumor Type: Breast cancer diagnosed 1975.
Treatment: Mastectomy.
Betty is the first non-gay spokesperson for the Human Rights Campaign's National Coming Out Project. Based in Washington, DC, they are the largest national gay and lesbian political organization, and they lobby for equal rights and fairness. Betty also writes a column for planitout.com with "mom advice" and is the author of the books "Love, Ellen: A mother Daughter Journey", and "Just a Mom."
Photo Credit: Anonymous.

JUST A MOM

You might imagine that Betty DeGeneres' biggest challenge was supporting her daughter's nationally televised coming-out party. Think again.

Twenty-five years ago, she entered a surgical procedure for a supposedly benign tumor, only to emerge without a breast.

"The doctor's report stated, 'To our surprise and chagrin, the report came back as malignant'." Betty adds, "No one was more surprised and chagrinned than I was that while I was under anesthesia, he performed the mastectomy."

After she recovered from the procedure—and the shock—she went about her life, hoping to make the "five-year" survival mark, getting back into yoga and strengthening her arm so that she could resume playing golf. In retrospect, Betty feels that she didn't allow herself proper time to heal physically and emotionally.

"I had surgery on Friday, came home on Monday, stayed at home on Tuesday and went back to work on Wednesday," she remembers. Nevertheless, she had a total recovery and didn't pursue reconstructive surgery, which wasn't nearly as common at the time as it is today.

A few years later, after turning fifty, she went back to college and received her Bachelor and Master's Degrees in speech pathology, a field she worked in for twelve years.

More than a mother, speech pathologist or emerging clinical psychologist, Betty defines herself these days as a "late-blooming activist." "Cancer makes you rethink your priorities," she says. "It made me realize the superficiality and commercialism of our world, depicted in the mass media by all the beautiful people and the beautiful bodies."

Following her daughter's public admission of her homosexuality, Betty became the first heterosexual spokesperson for the Human Rights Campaign's National Coming Out Campaign. "The organization does such a wonderful job in its mission," she reflects. "This work has been such a blessing in my life and has served as such a huge awakening to the need to accept diversity in all of its forms. Especially as parents, we need to love our children unconditionally."

She has also reconnected with her cancer experience in the past decade, participating in a recovery group for women who have had mastectomies. "Although mine was 15 years earlier, I never allowed myself to go through the grieving process, which I finally did through this group at my Episcopal Church."

Despite her cancer occurring a quarter-century ago, the positive effect it has had on her life remains. "I wake up and say, 'Thank you for this day!' every day," Betty offered.

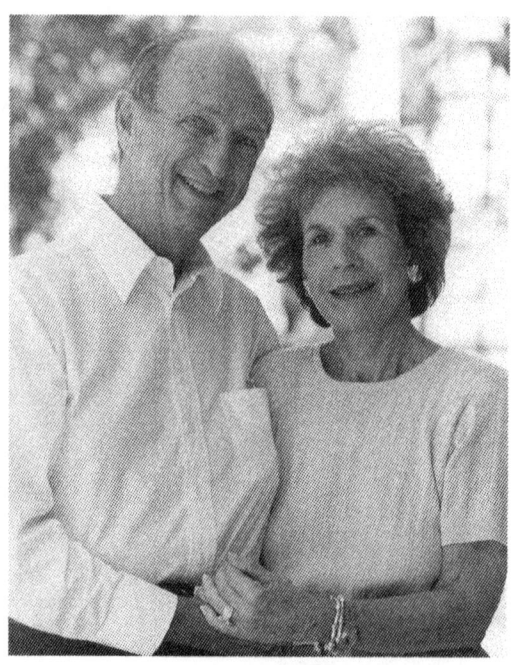

Richard Bloch, 74

Married 54 years to Annette, with 3 daughters and 7 grandchildren.
Richard and his brother Henry founded the tax-preparation company "H&R Block, Inc." He was chairman of the board until he retired in 1982.
Born: Kansas City, MO; Live: Kansas City, MO.
Tumor Type: Non Small Cell Lung Cancer diagnosed 1978.
Treatment: Radiation, Chemotherapy, Surgery (right lung removed) and Immunotherapy.
Richard and Annette fund many organizations, and the details of all that is available for free can be found on the web at *www.blastcancer.org*, and also at blochcancer.org. Their hotline offers free guides and a lot more, at 1-800-433-0464.
Photo Credit: Bloch Cancer Center. Picture taken with wife, Annette, at the Cancer Park in Kansas City, Missouri.

CANCER IS A WORD, NOT A SENTENCE

"I went from being told I had 90 days to live to being told I was cured—I could have flown home that day without an airplane."

These are the words of Richard Bloch, cofounder of H&R Block, Inc., the standard in American income tax preparation, and a lung cancer survivor.

By the time Richard was diagnosed, he had already been misdiagnosed twice. "At the time, I felt I was too young, too successful, too happy and had too good of a family to get cancer," Bloch remembers. "When another doctor finally diagnosed me, he said, 'You're a very sick boy, and we're going to have to make you a lot sicker before we can cure you. Then you can work to fight cancer.' He was true to his word."

The doctor told him to begin his therapy the next day in another city. After initially hesitating, his physician taught him the importance of making treatment a top priority in his life. "This doctor taught me more about cancer than anybody else I've ever met," Richard said. "He put together a team of doctors to treat me, because he said he didn't know enough, but was determined to beat it."

His first year of therapy was debilitating. "I was sick as a dog that first year—I looked like a 98-year-old man," Richard remarked. "But I kept it up and weathered the effects," he added. And the treatment—a combination of surgery, radiation and chemotherapy—was successful.

Years later, he entered a follow-up appointment hoping to hear that he was in remission. "I couldn't believe it when I was told that if my tumor type was gone for two years, the chance of it coming back is no greater than that of the man on the street."

After hearing the good news, Richard, like his doctor, was true to his word. Since his official "cure" in 1980, Richard and his wife, Annette, have devoted their lives to helping others with cancer beat the disease. He retired from H&R Block in 1992, and now considers cancer his life's work.

Among many other programs, the Bloch's have funded the development of more than 15 "Cancer Survivor Parks" across the United States, in which the beauty of nature complements statues and bronzed plaques that serve as inspiration for cancer patients.

"There are sculptures representing cancer and hope, among others, and a large maze representing cancer treatment," Richard described. "Someone who doesn't have cancer may have no interest in it, but in the cancer survivor or the newly diagnosed, it may subconsciously ignite their desire to fight rather than give up. If each park could somehow convince one or two people that it's worth the fight, then they've paid for themselves."

According to Richard, he and his wife will fund maintenance of the parks perpetually or "until there is no more cancer."

Richard is a living example of someone whose life was improved by cancer. "Recognition doesn't mean a thing," he remarked. "I'm working to help people now, instead of working for money. The greatest thrill of my life is to get my children and grandchildren together. That's all I want."

He also adds that his wife is his partner and is thankful for the many things she's done for him. "She says cancer is a word, not a sentence."

For those who can't visit his parks, Richard offers this advice: "The most important thing a newly diagnosed cancer patient can do is to make a commitment to themselves to do everything in their power to fight the disease. If they do that, they have no more decisions to make—everything else is automatic. As long as they put their health and their life first."

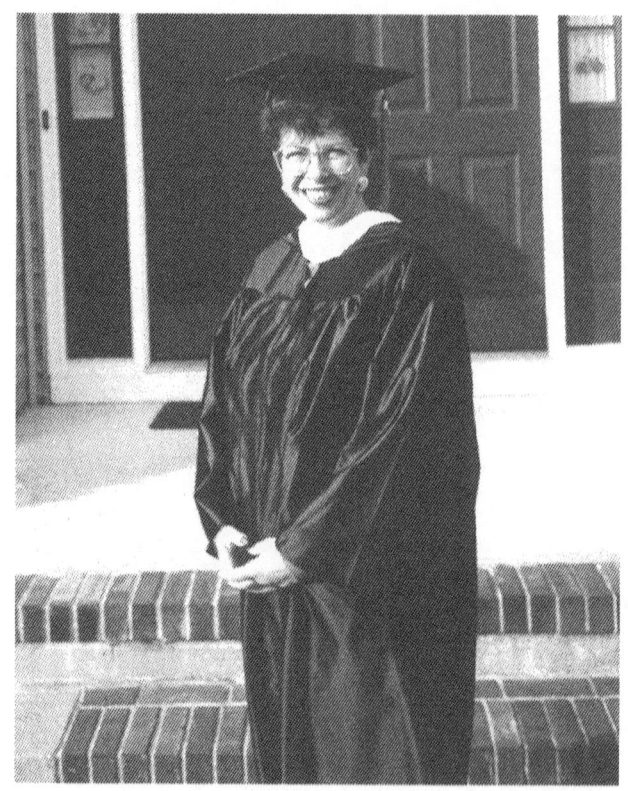

Camille Macchio, 50

Married 21 years to Robert, with one daughter (30).
Camille is a Communications Manager at Johnson and Johnson NCS.
Born: Brooklyn NY. Lives: Milltown NJ
Tumor Type: Hodgkin's Lymphoma (stage 2a) diagnosed 1995.
Treatment: Chemotherapy.
Camille supports Sloan Kettering Hospital in New York City.
Photo Credit: Robert Macchio.

THE COME-BACK KID

Her first potential indication that something had gone awry was a necklace that didn't lay flat on her chest. Her next recollection was a clump of hair in her hand.

"The minute that huge lock of hair fell out, I just couldn't believe it," expressed Camille Macchio, a Hodgkin's Lymphoma survivor. "I broke down."

Her emotional reaction came after months of remaining relatively calm throughout her diagnosis and treatment planning. "While I wasn't someone who would sit in the corner and lick my wounds, my initial reaction was one of nonreaction," Camille said.

She calmly dedicated herself to the task at hand—interviewing doctors, learning about her treatment options and researching clinical trials. "It's only when I was in the midst of chemo that the reality of what I was going through began to hit home," Camille recalls.

She started to feel better when she was able to appreciate the comic relief of her own situation. "I happen to have a very small head, so I had to go to the children's department to find a hat," Camille said. She and her husband laughed about it. Not long after, her hair began to grow back, but she also began to experience severe side effects from chemotherapy.

Through it all, Camille continued to exercise at the gym. "Your whole 24-hour-a-day existence doesn't have to be chemo," she advises. "I did my chemo, I worked out at the gym and went out on weekends. I never had a better appetite, despite the metallic taste in my mouth the chemo caused; even when nothing tasted good, I ate anyway," Camille says with a laugh.

Camille learned to focus more on herself during her cancer experience. "Concentrate on you," she advises. "Find people who support you, don't worry about those who are uncomfortable about your situation and realize that you may need to train people in how to treat you."

Her mother and daughter did not react well to her physical state during chemotherapy, and she banned her husband from accompanying her to one chemotherapy session because "he looked at me with those big doggy brown eyes and I could tell he was feeling sorry for me," she described.

There was a point when she tired of wearing a wig and threw it on her seat at a gas station. "The attendant thought it was a cat, and I told him it was a wig. He said I didn't need one. I never wore it again."

Part of concentrating on yourself, Camille says, is being aware of the effects of your disease beyond the cancer. "You have to consider the psychological and physical effects of someone in our situation, like early menopause or the effects of radiation on your dental health," she remarked. "You still have to think of your life 20 years down the road," Camille added.

Focusing on her own recovery helped her to be more forgiving of her own and others' shortcomings. "I now realize that just because I can't do something today, it's not a sign of weakness or inability, perhaps just due to the fact that I don't have that particular skill set," she explained. "I'm more apt to give others a break, too, because I realize that I might not really know what they're going through."

Cancer-free five years later, Camille is "so thrilled about all of the little things." The May after her last treatment, she completed her Bachelor's degree and was promoted from an administrative to a managerial position with her company. She also now enjoys photography because now when she looks through the lens, she sees things differently.

And she no longer sweats the small stuff. "Rain doesn't bother me anymore—it's just water," Camille remarked. In her work with Cancer Care, Inc., a cancer support organization, she has signed up to be a buddy for newly diagnosed Hodgkin's Lymphoma patients. "My life has changed and I'd like to help to change others' lives around me."

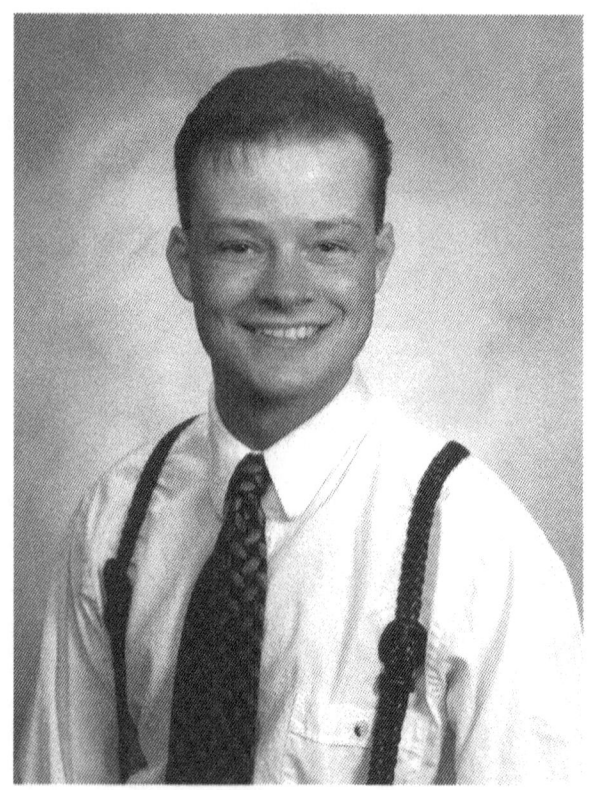

Eric Waldon, 27

Single.
Eric is a full time student in a Masters of Music Therapy and Masters in Counseling Psychology program.
Born: Dayton, OH. Lives: Stockton, CA
Tumor Type: Lymphocytic ('child') Leukemia, diagnosed February 1993.
Treatment: Chemotherapy and an autologous (self) peripheral stem cell transplant. Prophylactic chemotherapy injected into the spine to help prevent metastases.
Photo Credit: Unknown

I MAY NOT BE WHAT I OUGHT TO BE BUT I SURE AIN'T WHAT I USED TO BE

"When I was told I had leukemia, I almost fell off my chair," reports 27-year-old Eric Waldon. "I was scared of the uncertainly—but thankful that I wasn't dead."

His diagnosis came after reporting "mono-like" symptoms to his doctor during the summer after his junior year in college. The events that followed all happened so fast that Eric didn't even have time to call and tell his friends.

"That Friday, which happened to be Friday the 13, I went to my general practitioner, who referred me to an internist, who then referred me to an oncologist," Eric recalls. "By one o'clock in the afternoon, I was admitted into the hospital and had the bone marrow aspiration and surgery to insert a subcutaneous central line and a hemodialysis catheter."

He received prophylactic chemotherapy into his spinal fluid to prevent metastases, donated and underwent a transplant of his own bone marrow and had high-dose chemotherapy as a preventive measure against further disease. Eric achieved remission during his first three weeks in the hospital and has never relapsed. "My doctors were actually surprised at how well I responded," he says.

Eric took the next year off school, referring to it as his "sabbatical," and then re-entered Western Michigan University, changing his major from music education to music therapy, "for obvious reasons," he reports. "I thought about going into medicine, but I don't like medicine," Eric laughs. "Music was my first love, and music therapy just seemed like the perfect solution—using my music to help others with cancer."

He now is in the Masters of Music Therapy and Masters in Counseling Psychology program. "My particular interest is working with cancer patients and others to train them to use music to relax and as a means of distracting them from painful or negative stimuli," Eric explained. "Music therapy can also make it easier for people to express their feelings and emotions."

As he now can. Since his diagnosis, Eric reports being more forgiving, empathetic and less self-focused. It has also afforded him the opportunity to reestablish his relationship with his father, with whom he was never really close since his parents' divorce when he was a young child.

"Cancer has given me the license to do all of these things," Eric remarked.

"Now I can take some risk, be more adventurous and live life to its fullest."

During treatment, Eric stayed with a woman in the community near the hospital, who often served as his sounding board at the end of the day. He said that she told him a line from a song that summarizes his life after cancer and the prospect of getting better every year: "I may not be what I ought to be, but I sure ain't what I used to be."

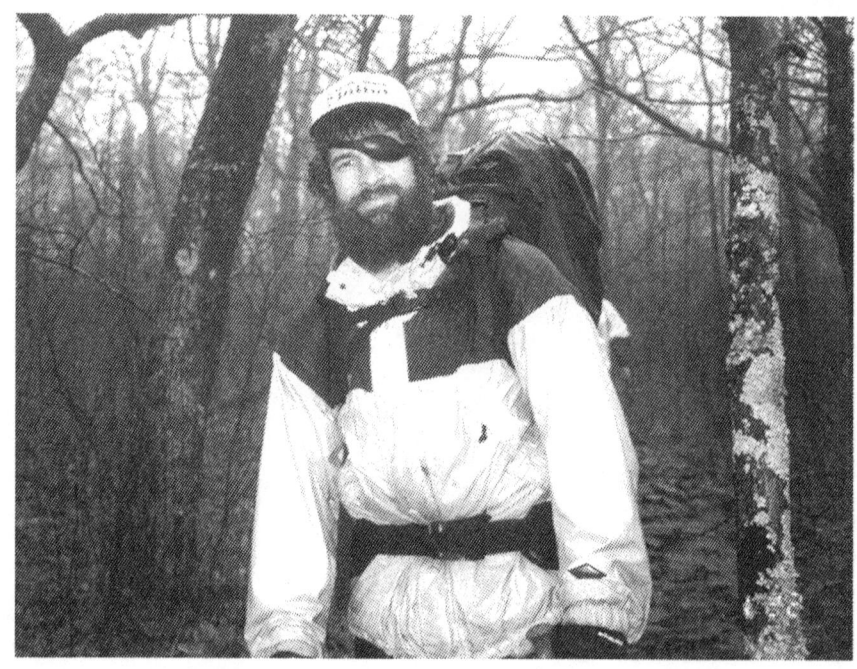

Jay Platt, 35

Married three years to Paz.

Jay, a retired Marine Corps Gunnery Sergeant, is a professional speaker and the author of 'A Time to Walk: Life Lessons Learned on the Appalachian Trail.' He can be reached on the web at www.jayplatt.com.

Born: Quitman, GA. Lives: Cartersville GA.

Tumor Type: von Hippel Lindau (VHL) Syndrome, with tumors in the eye, brain, spine and kidneys diagnosed 1986. For more info on VHL, please visit www.vhl.org.

Treatment: Ten surgeries to remove tumors.

Photo Credit: Unknown. Photo taken on the last day of his hike through the entire Appalachian Trail.

WAHOO, I MADE IT

If surviving cancer were a lot like hiking the Appalachian Trail, then Jay Platt would know.

He recently finished hiking the 2,160-mile Trail to raise money for the von Hippel Lindau Family Alliance. "Hiking for cancer gave me a great motive, since you have to average about 15 miles a day with a heavy pack," Jay explained. In addition, he hiked the trail the opposite direction that most people do—from Maine to Georgia—experiencing much rougher terrain and also loneliness, since his colleagues were hiking in the opposite direction. He wanted the extra challenge.

Jay completed the trek in five and a half months and it was "much, much harder than I originally anticipated—I lost 25 pounds in the process." In the end, he was successful in completing the journey and helped raise $109,000 for the cause.

Jay was originally diagnosed in 1986 when he was having black wavy lines in his vision. Subsequently, surgeons removed his left eye and also his left testicle, thinking it was also cancerous. In the end, it was not.

In 1995, things took a turn for the worse, when a checkup discovered suspicious-looking tumors on his left kidney. Once they were determined to be malignant, he was sent to Bethesda Naval Hospital, since he was in the Marines at the time. While the original plan was to remove the tumors in his kidney, Jay mentioned to the doctors that he had been having terrible headaches and dizziness.

Following further tests, four tumors were found in his brain. Jay underwent an 11-hour brain surgery to remove three of the tumors, but the fourth couldn't be reached. Following a month of recovery, he underwent the removal of a portion of his kidney. Since then, more tumors have been discovered on his spinal cord, other kidney and brain, but have not grown enough for surgery. Jay is currently in a "wait and see" situation.

While the news of the additional tumors was a severe blow, Jay decided to draw from the discipline he gained in his Marine training to fight his new enemy. "I realized that I could either go home, become a couch potato and just fade away, or I could do something to show myself and the world that I wasn't down for the count," he said. "I dug my heels in and said, 'I'm going to fight this thing.'"

Not long after, he read the story of Terry Fox, a Canadian who lost his leg to cancer and ran across his native country to raise money for cancer. Unfortunately, he died during his journey, but his story has inspired many of his followers, including Jay, who then decided to embark on the Appalachian Trail adventure. Along the trail, every fifteen miles, there's a register to sign in on. Jay contemplated the words of wisdom he'd write. On the last day, he settled on 'Wahoo, I made it'. "It was lame and I knew it, but it was enough."

While things are still somewhat uncertain, Jay reports "feeling fantastic. When I was first diagnosed, my initial thought was, 'Why me?' Now I know that if I hadn't gone through cancer, I wouldn't be the same person I am today."

Had his Marine training prepared him for the mental fight he's undergone? "When you deal with a disease like this for seven years, you become tough mentally because you realize that you can do anything," Jay reports. "Along the way, you come to realize that the winner is the one who doesn't give up. Perseverance pays off."

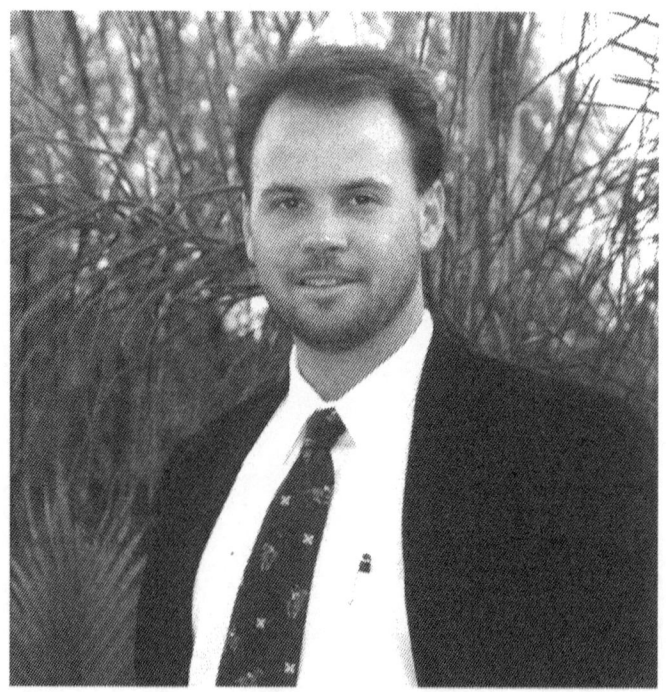

Dr. Corey Gonzales, 37

Married 6 years to Jamie.
Corey is a licensed Clinical Psychologist in private practice, dealing largely with cancer patients, and can be reached for speaking engagements through 661-834-8341.
Born: Concord, California. Live: Bakersfield, California.
Tumor Type: Testicular cancer diagnosed December 6, 1985. Metastases to the lungs.
Treatment: Orchiectomy (surgical removal of the affected testicle), removal of surrounding lymph nodes, and eight months of chemotherapy. Dr. Gonzales supports the American Cancer Society. To find therapy, call the ACS in your area or the main number toll-free at 1-800-4CANCER.
Photo Credit: Wife Jamie Gonzales for Coping Magazine.

FROM FEAR TO FOCUS

At the age of 23, he had an orchiectomy—surgical removal of the testicle—and didn't even know he had cancer.

Now 37, Dr. Corey Gonzales is a survivor whose life's work is counseling others battling the disease. "Being an active participant in your treatment is very important," he advises. "Get educated about what's going on, find a doctor you feel comfortable with and do research. The more you know about what you're dealing with, the more likely you'll be to experience less fear and anxiety. You'll find the situation more tolerable and feel a stronger sense of control."

Corey's cancer was discovered during a college baseball physical. His trainer discovered the lump and referred him to a urologist. He was admitted to the hospital for surgery that night. Chemotherapy began about a month later.

"The metastases to the lungs and lymph nodes were extensive, and my prognosis was terminal," Corey recounts. "The cancer shattered my hopes of becoming a professional baseball player—I hit .340 the year before and was hoping to be signed by the San Francisco Giants the next year."

Corey officially discovered that he had cancer after his surgery, when a doctor came into the room and introduced himself as an oncologist. "I asked him what that was—I heard that I had a tumor, but didn't even know that I had cancer when I had the orchiectomy," he said.

He broke down crying and asked his doctor if he was going to die. "He answered, 'Yes, there is a chance,' but said the odds were in my favor because of my age, health and physical strength." Afterwards, he remembers the specialist saying, "I'm going to go after this very aggressively and I think we can get it if you're ready to battle." Corey added, "We shook hands and I knew he cared about my well-being. I felt like we were partners and that was very important to me."

While in treatment, Corey completed his Master's Degree and moved from San Francisco to Los Angeles to begin his Doctorate. That's when his official training in clinical psychiatry began. He began working with young adults with cancer through an organization called "Vital Options" (*See Selma Shimmell's story.*)

"The issues that young people with cancer face are different from someone in their 50s or 60s," Corey explained. "Young adults have unique issues, like young female breast cancer patients who have body image issues, concerns about finding a partner and concerns about their future fertility."

Corey adds that, in his own life, fertility is an issue, "but fortunately I have a wife who's okay with that. We don't feel the need to have children to make this a valid marriage."

Corey also helped initiate the first "Man-to-Man" program in California for men with prostate cancer, while working as a psychiatric assistant pursuing his license. "After cancer, you need to heal. You need to look at the scars, make amends with your body and begin to feel comfortable with yourself again," he expressed.

In counseling his patients on taking control of their cancer experience, he recounts his own chemotherapy experience. "When I started losing my hair, I felt like a victim watching it come out in clumps in the shower and on my pillow," Corey recalled. "Finally, my dad, brother and I got together and just shaved it off."

Like treatment side effects, Corey said that life itself is only temporary. "We need to understand that all of us will die at some point," he said. "Either you're alive or you're dead—there's no in-between. Cancer makes us do an inventory of our lives so that we can see what's important and begin to embrace every moment."

Corey is still an avid baseball fan. He runs three to four miles every morning, plays golf on Fridays, tries to manage his stress and takes daily vitamins.

As a patient and counselor, he emphasizes the importance of not going through cancer alone. "When you go through a life-threatening illness it's considered a trauma," Corey explained. "It's normal to feel stress, anxiety and depression, which is why it's so critical that you're supported by other people who are going through similar experiences so that you don't feel so 'crazy.'"

As you're going through cancer, Corey says to keep your sights on the silver lining. "Don't ever give up hope and never relinquish your goals," he said. "You need to hang onto something that keeps you moving forward and growing—something that continues to give your life meaning."

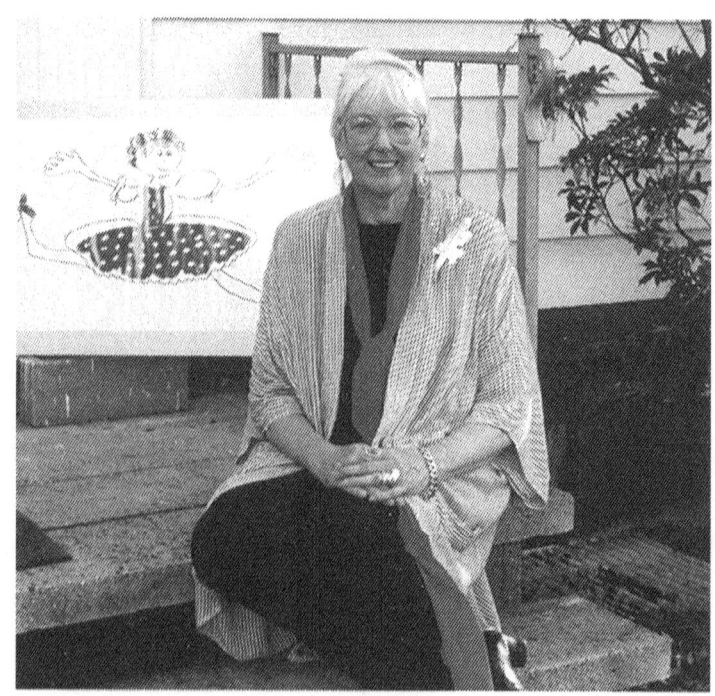

Anne Wennhold, 67

Widowed since 1969, no children. "I borrow my brother's"
Anne is retired but working part time for various county agencies, as a facilitator for drug and alcohol outpatients and senior citizens. She worked for a hospital's public relations department for 17 years as a photographer.
Born: St. Louis, MO. Lives: Leonia, NJ
Tumor Type: Breast Cancer diagnosed February 1989.
Treatment: Chemotherapy and Mastectomy.
Photo Credit: Kathy Rebek

JOURNEY TOWARD HEALING

Becoming an advocate for your own health care is not uncommon in cancer care—telling your surgeon to wake you up during your surgery to give you your pathology results is something else.

But not for 67-year-old Anne Wennhold, a breast cancer survivor who recalls feeling angry when a plastic surgeon told her that she should opt to have an implant during her surgery. Anne wanted to decide based on the results of her surgery.

"The plastic surgeon said, 'You really don't know what you want. You should do it and you'll thank me afterwards,'" Anne recalls. "I was really, really angry that he thought I couldn't make the decision myself. I just wanted the right to choose."

To ensure that the choice was indeed hers, Anne directed her surgeon to wake her up during the lumpectomy to update her on the results of the pathology report. Concurrently, the surgeon reported that they were going to proceed with the mastectomy. She decided not to receive the implant.

Afterwards, her primary surgeon told her that she had a 90+ percent chance of recovery because her tumor was encapsulated. "He told me to get back to living my life," Anne remarked. Easier said than done.

Anne became depressed and her physician referred her to a therapist, who used art therapy to aid her in her emotional recovery. She began drawing and coloring—activities she enjoyed in childhood—and end up creating a 150-foot-long mural at the end of nine months.

"Art therapy enabled me to escape into another world, to get my feelings out and to express in pictures what I wasn't able to express in words," Anne explains. "It unlocked a cascade of feelings that I had set aside while putting my energy into physical recovery."

Raised not to complain or to openly express sadness or anger, Anne now knows that emotions are a very important aspect of the total being. "I tell people that you must deal with the emotions of illness or crisis in order to be able to move past the experience and to get on with your life."

A photographer by trade, she created a slide show of her mural piece by piece and presented it to local groups, including the New Jersey chapter of the American Cancer Society and support groups throughout the tri-state area.

When asked to talk with newly diagnosed patients, Anne never offers advice. She sits down with the women and asks them to talk about the options and how they feel about them. She does, however, suggest that they "do something you enjoy so much you forget about the illness, even momentarily. That is one way to help yourself toward healing from the beginning of the diagnosis."

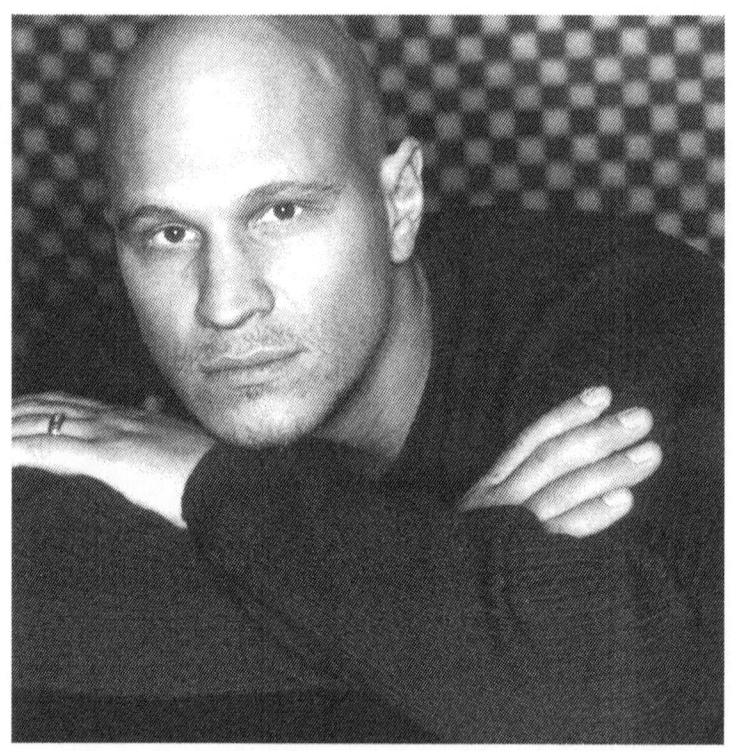

Kevin Sharp, 29

Married 2 years to Tracy.
Recording artist/entertainer.
Born: Reading, CA; Live: Springhill, TN.
Tumor Type: Ewing's Sarcoma of the left femur (thighbone) and hip, diagnosed August 1989. Metastases to lungs.
Treatment: Surgeries, Chemotherapy and Radiation.
Kevin has two CD's, "Measure of a Man" and "Love Is." He is working on a third CD and a book about his experiences. He supports the Make-A-Wish Foundation and the American Cancer Society. Find out more at www.kevinsharp.com
Photo Credit—Nancy Lee Andrews.

LOVE ONE ANOTHER

While most 18-year-old teens are concerned about dates, cars and college, Kevin Sharp's recollection of this year of his life is one of non-stop chemotherapy.

"Lying in the hospital at night, every minute seems like an hour," Kevin recalls. "It gives you time to do an incredible amount of soul-searching, which is when I decided to quit asking, 'Why me?'"

Despite being raised in a very devout family, and living a healthy lifestyle, Kevin initially felt that his diagnosis of cancer was a punishment from God. "It took me awhile to realize that God wasn't punishing me for some mistake in my life. I went from thinking, "Why me?' to "Why not me?' and decided to do something positive with my life."

Following his diagnosis of Ewing's Sarcoma, Kevin underwent surgery, chemotherapy and radiation. He broke his leg, a side effect of radiation, which lead to the discovery that the chemo wasn't working.

"We started again from scratch," Kevin said, "and entered a much more aggressive therapy for a week each month for over a year." Following chemo and surgery to repair broken bones, he was told that the cancer was expected to recur within two months. Nearly 10 years later, he remains cancer-free.

Battling cancer at such a young age, he admits that there were some cloudy days, as there still are. "The main thing is to stay focused and do everything in your personal power to make what's tough in your life into a positive lesson," he said. He now schools others in his lessons through talking with children with cancer in the hospital and becoming involved in local charities.

A large part of his advice is telling people to take care of themselves and get the right support. "Doctors aren't perfect," Kevin purports. "A good doctor is a real person who listens to you and understands that every person is different. If you find a doctor who tells you that he knows everything about your cancer, you better turn and run away!" Kevin also made a point of praising the role of nurses in caring and providing emotional support for cancer patients.

Kevin also sings the praises in song. Through the charity of the "Make-a-Wish Foundation," he met his idol, David Foster, and he spends a great deal of time returning the favor to the Foundation. Since, he has recorded two CDs and is writing a book about his experience with cancer.

"Music is such a powerful tool in everyday life," Kevin believes. "It can even help people through the most trying times in their lives. It's not about money, or how many things you collect, it's about what you give back, and how much you care about the person standing next to you." When Kevin thinks about the most important lesson he wants to share, he says without hesitation "just love one another."

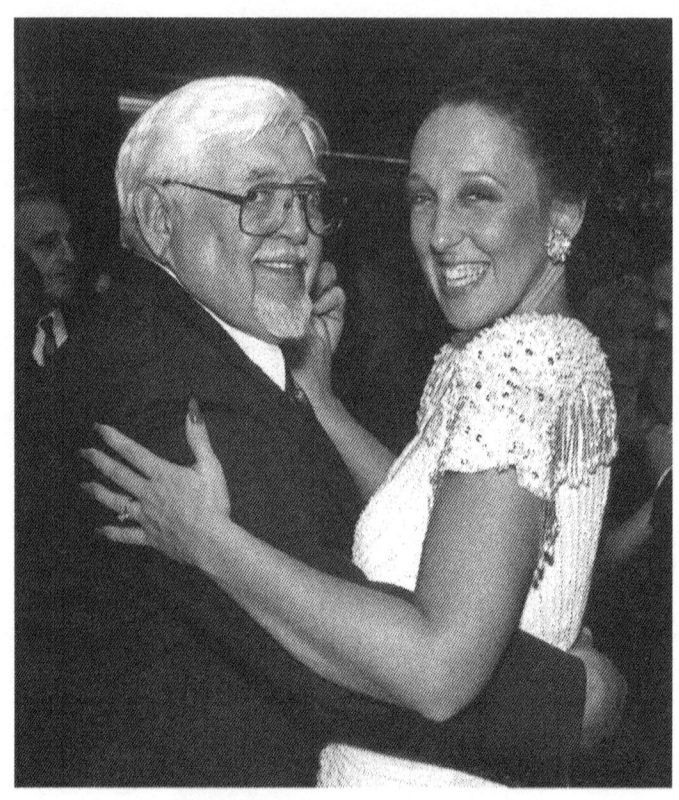

Suzanne Guimond Wilson, 44

Married 21 years with daughter Jenny (16) and son Michael (12).
Suzanne is the administrative director of medical education at Mount Clemens General Hospital in Mt. Clemens, Michigan.
Born: Detroit, MI. Lives: Great Lakes area.
Tumor Type: Cervical neuroblastoma (nerve tumor in the neck) diagnosed at age 2 and metastatic thyroid cancer at age 13.
Treatment: Radiation for the neuroblastoma, resulting in metastatic thyroid cancer at age 13. Thyroid removed.
Photo Credit: Unknown, with her father, who has since died.

THE BADGE OF COURAGE

Suzanne Guimond Wilson's earliest recollection of undergoing radiation treatments alone at the age of two was that she really wasn't alone—her stuffed tiger was her constant companion.

"I still remember being alone in the room without my parents and having the big machine over me making noise," Suzanne vividly remembers. "It was so frightening for a kid."

To calm her fears, her grandfather gave her a stuffed tiger "that he said would protect me and keep me safe," she said. "Being only two, I believed his every word and my tiger helped me get through those treatments." Incidentally, the tiger is still very much with her, albeit missing one eye. "His fur has been very much loved off, but he's still around." And so is Suzanne, four decades later, despite another recurrence when she was 13.

Her cancer spread to both sides of her neck, and Suzanne's lymph nodes were taken out on both sides. The surgery was very disfiguring and left her badly scarred. "At 13, you're just developing your own identity. I felt like Frankenstein's monster," she said. "Not only that, I honestly didn't think I was going to survive."

But she did, and has remained cancer-free since. While Suzanne's physical scars remain, the emotional ones began to abate, aided with the passage of time and maturity.

"You begin to accept that this is who you are," she said. "I consider my scars a badge of honor. They show that I've fought some pretty serious battles—and won."

Suzanne received her Bachelor's and Master's degrees in nursing, and has been active in accreditation of nursing continuing education, as well as changing practices for the selection of interns in her hospital by assessing a number of more nonconventional competencies, such as compassion, teamwork and communications skills.

She is active in cancer support organizations, such as the National Cancer Survivor's Day speaker's bureau, and considers herself an "extreme gardener". With such a busy professional and personal life, does she think about her cancer?

"Being a cancer survivor is analogous to having a background task running on your computer while you're working on something else," Suzanne explained. "It's always there, but you don't always pay a lot of attention to it. Once in a while, you may have a scare, and it can be depressing and preoccupying. But you just have to keep putting one foot in front of the other and keep walking along until you make sure you're safe again."

Like many of us, Suzanne is still working on her ability to fully stop and smell the roses, along with her husband and teenage children. "I think of my life as still evolving," she says. "I try to be a good person and do the right thing. I would like to believe I've done some good things that will be remembered by the people who love me after I'm gone."

She adds, "No matter what happens, you have to have hope. The most fatal thing you can face isn't the cancer itself; it's a loss of hope. Look at me—I did all right."

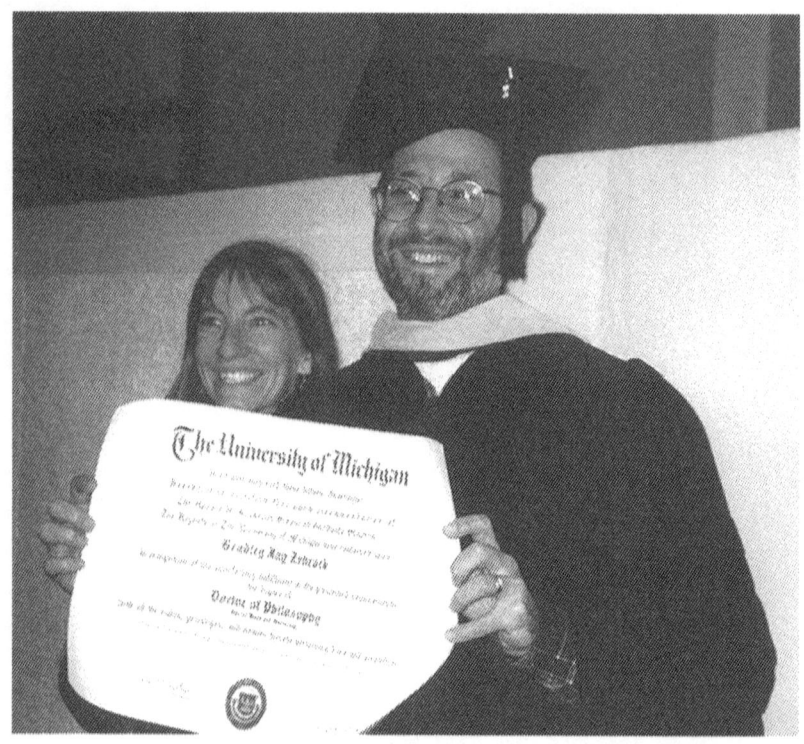
Brad Zebrack, 40

Married 11 years to Joanne, "no children yet".
Brad is a Research Fellow at the UCLA Cancer Center, researching the quality of life of long term survivors of cancer.
Born: North Hollywood, CA. Lives: Los Angeles, CA
Tumor Type: Hodgkin's Disease diagnosed in 1985 at age 25.
Treatment: Chemotherapy.
Brad supports the National Coalition for Cancer Survivorship, who his "Ride For Survivorship" was dedicated to. They also do great work for current and future cancer survivors, regarding health care, support, and a whole lot more.
Photo Credit—Melanie Holcomb.

RIDE FOR SURVIVORSHIP

After completing treatment for Hodgkin's Disease, most people resume work and refocus on their hobbies and loved ones. Not Brad Zebrack—he embarked on an 11,000-mile bike ride around the perimeter of the United States.

"When my doctors told me that I had to put my life on hold for a year to undergo treatment, I decided that I would like to do something exciting for the next year after it was all over," Brad explained. So he and Joanne set off on their bikes for a year.

Always an avid cyclist, Brad unknowingly began to experience cancer symptoms on an earlier 3,000-mike trek from San Francisco to Boston, including night sweats, itching and a lump on his neck. His father, a physician, saw the lump and referred him to an oncologist. His dad was also the bearer of Brad's bad news.

Following Brad's diagnosis at the age of 25, chemotherapy took its toll on him. "I got more sick after each cycle and it took me longer to bounce back from each one," Brad recalls. He survived treatment, which ended in late 1986, and began writing to magazines for counsel on how to plan his trip around the U.S.

"People all over the country wrote to us pledging their emotional and financial support, and by June of 1988 our friends met us for a big send-off party," Brad remembers.

He described his itinerary: "We went north (toward Washington State), across the northern states during the summer and arrived in Maine by fall. Then we headed down the Atlantic coast to Florida, arriving by winter, and then rode back across the southern states during the spring. We made it back to California in the summer of 1989."

Brad's bike ride with his girlfriend, Joanne, encompassed 11,000 miles in total. "After the trip we got married," he reports.

Upon returning, he has shared his experiences with others at hospitals and treatment centers around the country through work with the National Coalition for Cancer Survivorship (NCCS). "My hope was that if young people could see me riding my bike around the country, they too could understand that survivorship is possible," Brad said. "Being a role model for other cancer patients was my driving force every mile of the trip."

This goal has also been the driving force in his career. Brad is currently a Research Fellow at the UCLA Cancer Center, where he is involved in scientific investigation into the quality of life of long-term cancer survivors.

It doesn't take too much scientific study to realize that Brad's quality of life is just fine. He and Joanne are pursuing adoption of a child; he became sterile as a result of chemotherapy. He has also taken up "long stitch," a sort of paint-by-numbers with yarn of different colors, recently using the technique to create a baby gift for his sister.

One thing he doesn't do now: watch television newscasts.

"I find that it's such a warped presentation of the world we live in," he prophesizes. "For every bad thing that happens, there are probably 10 more good things that you don't hear about. It would be like me reporting on my cycling trip and making a point to tell you that someone once threw an apple at us, rather than discussing the incredible generosity and outpourings of kindness we experienced."

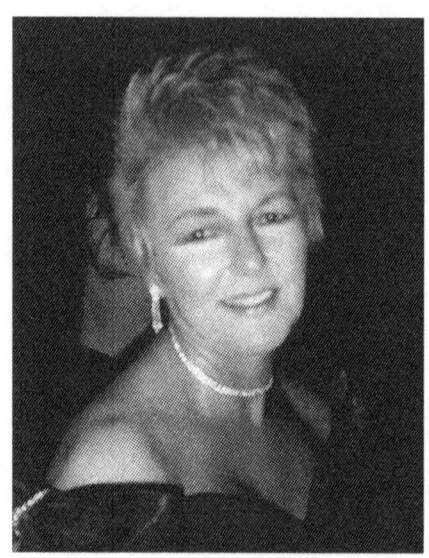

Jan Harris, 55

Single, with sons 21 and 25.

Jan is the Director of the Angel Care Breast Cancer Foundation (angelcarefoundation.org), a non-profit organization comprised of breast cancer survivors who will accompany any woman in the Redmond, Washington area to breast cancer care, support and follow-up appointments. They are at 17125 Northeast 98th Court, Redmond, Washington 98052 and can be emailed at angelcare3@aol.com. Their funding comes from private grants, and they are a United Way agency. Their number is 425-861-5655.

Born: Seattle, WA. Live: Redmond, WA (a suburb of Seattle).

Tumor Type: Breast cancer (stage 3) diagnosed 1993, spread to 18 lymph nodes.

Treatment: Mastectomy, chemotherapy, radiation, and five years of Tamoxifen therapy. First mastectomy followed by a prophylactic (optional) second mastectomy.

Photo Credit: Unknown. Taken on cruise vacation just two months after reconstructive surgery.

ANGEL ON A MISSION

Jan Harris' advice to cancer patients is to hang out with upbeat people.

At the age of 55, she has survived Stage 3 breast cancer with involvement in 18 lymph nodes. "There's no magic," Jan says. "Eat well, go out and live a pretty normal life like you did before. And remember to laugh."

That's the advice she gives through her agency, the Angel Care Foundation. "We instill in people we work with that people do get through treatments, they live and they can have quality of life," she remarked.

Jan was diagnosed in 1993 and underwent a mastectomy, chemotherapy, radiation and five years of Tamoxifen. "I had a 30% chance of living five years," she remarked. "I'd be lying if I said it was easy. I feel in my heart that God had another plan for me; maybe He said, 'I'll save her because I want her to do something else to reach out and help others.'"

Jan had reconstructive surgery after her first mastectomy. Being a single mom "and living being a high priority," she opted to have a second prophylactic mastectomy and an implant. "I said God gave me a second chance, so I picked the size I wanted the second time around. I told that doctor that I was opting for cleavage this time and I want to have nice firm breasts even when I'm into my 90s."

As you can tell, humor for Jan was a wonderful healer. "My doctor would ask me what I've done for fun," Jan recalls. "In the beginning, I thought, 'Fun, what fun? I've got cancer." But he'd ask me the same question every single week.

Tired of not having a suitable answer, Jan starting going out with friends to see a movies and would dress up to feel good. "After awhile, I started going to chemo wearing bright, flashy colors, and I bought a gold hat with a big brim on it in the spring, which I even wore to chemo," she noted. "I wanted my children to see me as a mother that looked healthy instead of a mother that looked like she was going to die."

As part of their services, Angel Care volunteers accompany women to help them shop for a wig. "We don't just get the wig, we make it a pleasurable outing," Jan reports. "We go for coffee or tea or something afterwards, and do the same thing with a prosthesis—a lot of women are embarrassed to ask a friend or their husband to go with them."

She also engages perfect strangers in discussing their cancer experience. "When I see someone with no hair and no eyebrows, I'll approach them and compliment them on their haircut, saying, 'Hey, I had a hairdo like that for a year.'" She said that before she knows it, the person is asking her about her chemo and "you find yourself hugging this perfect stranger in the vegetable department in the grocery store, knowing that seeing you alive years later has given them hope. When someone brightens up because you've given them hope, it makes us stronger as a result."

Jan says that information sharing is key to recovery. "You can't just show up and expect the doctor to have all the magic," she advises. "Nor can you expect God to save you out of pity. He's a busy person; that's why he gave us brains. Don't let emotions make your choices for you."

The idea for Angel Care came to her while reading a newspaper one evening, and she left her job at a bank to get started. "The organization gave me a mission in life, a reason to live," she said. "We need a reason to get up in the morning and do something that makes a difference for others in order to rekindle our fighting spirit."

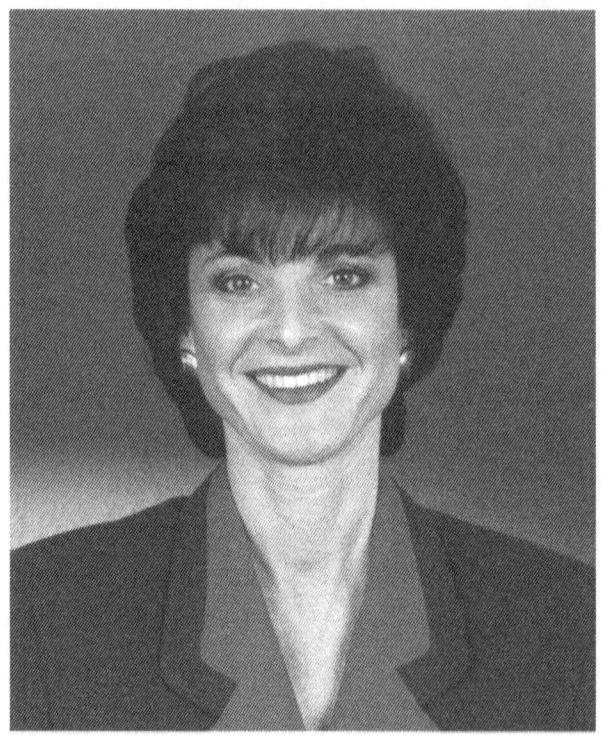

Christine Clifford, 47

Married 26 years to John, with sons Tim 17 and Brooks 14.
Christine is the CEO and President of The Cancer Club (www.cancerclub.com) and a professional speaker and author. The Cancer Club has a quarterly newsletter featuring humorous articles and helpful products or information. They also sell books, audiocassettes, videotapes, computer software, custom jewelry, T-shirts, and over 30 different items. Her company's trademarked motto is "Don't Forget to Laugh!"
Born: St. Claire Shores, MI. Live: Edina, MN.
Tumor Type: Breast Cancer (grade 3) diagnosed December 1994.
Treatment: Lumpectomy followed by chemotherapy and radiation.
Photo Credit: John Michael Kearney

DON'T FORGET TO LAUGH!™

Having a mother die of breast cancer at an early age and receiving a diagnosis of breast cancer herself, it's hard to believe that Christine Clifford could find humor in the situation.

"My mother died of breast cancer in her early '40s, after a horrible illness," she recounts. "My immediate reaction to my diagnosis was, 'I'm going to die.'"

Early in her treatment process—a lumpectomy, chemotherapy and radiation—Christine began to experience the positive side effects of humor. "Not only did humor connect people and put them at ease, I found it to be a very healing method of dealing with my cancer," she remarked.

Four weeks after her diagnosis, Christine said she entered the "Twilight Zone." "I woke up in the middle of the night and went downstairs into our family room and sketched over 50 cartoons of what had happened to me up to that point," Christine remembers. "Before that, I had never drawn, had never written a book and hadn't considered myself a particularly humorous person."

The next day, she got up and queried local librarians and bookstore clerks about the availability of humorous books about cancer. "Little did I know at the time that their reactions—including one person who said, 'Cartoons about cancer? You're sick!'—would be the basis for a book, let alone a support organization and an entire company!"

"From then on, I sought out and chronicled humor in every situation in my cancer experience, and began to use the cartoons on thank you cards that I sent to friends and well-wishers," she added.

On the one-year anniversary of her surgery, Christine signed a contract to publish not one, but two, books: *Not Now... I'm Having a No Hair Day!* and *Our Family Has Cancer, Too*. She has since written *Inspiring*

Breakthrough Secrets to Live Your Dreams and *Cancer Has Its Privileges: Stories of Hope & Laughter.*

Publication of her books spurred Christine to quit her high-stress position as a senior executive in marketing. "My job had not only been stressful, but also time consuming and not necessarily enjoyable," she said. "Now, my work is more like a hobby."

In the past six years, she has also quit smoking, started lifting weights, walking, playing golf and skiing. "The biggest life change I made was my ability to start focusing on the fun in life instead of all of the seriousness."

She also has lofty goals of giving back to the community, and founded *The Christine Clifford Celebrity Golf Invitational,* which has raised over $500,000 for breast cancer research in three years.

In addition to good medical care, Christine advises the newly diagnosed to research all of the possibilities, ask for help and, most of all, "Don't forget to laugh!"™

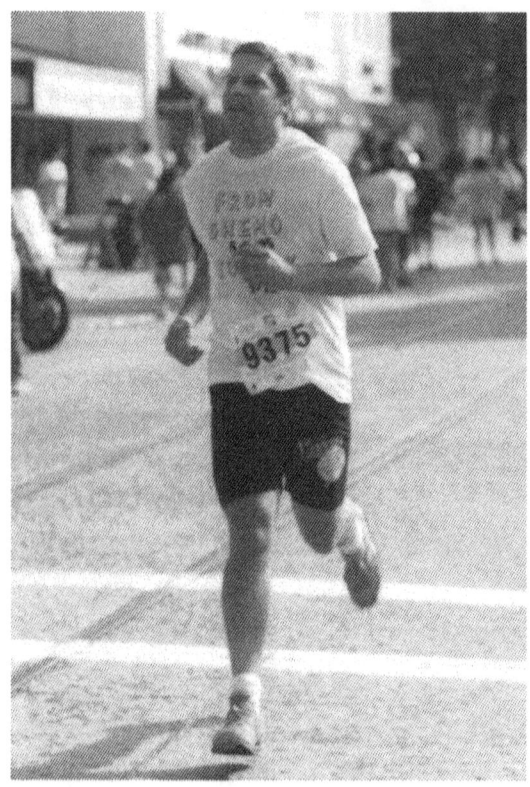

Geoffrey Nance, 42

Single. Lives with his son, 15, and girlfriend, Yvonne Johnson.
Geoffrey is a financial advisor and a licensed securities broker (for stocks, bonds, and mutual funds) for Prudential Securities.
Born: Glen Cove, NY. Lives: East Northport, NY.
Tumor Type: Stage 3 Non-Hodgkin's Lymphoma diagnosed November 1994 with two recurrences.
Treatment: Chemotherapy. Stem Cell replacement procedure done for second diagnosis with high-dosage chemotherapy. Third diagnosis, gene-targeted chemo with radiation.
Photo Credit: Island Photography. On Great Cow Harbor Run.

STRONG LIKE BULL

Visualization and being "strong like bull" helped Geoffrey Nance weather his very intensive and aggressive treatments for Non-Hodgkin's Lymphoma.

Following his initial diagnosis, he underwent chemotherapy. Following his second, he had a stem cell replacement with high-dose chemotherapy. After his third, he was given a gene-targeted chemotherapy regimen with radiation.

"A doctor once told me that I had a very strong constitution, and that's one of the reasons I believe I made it through all of the procedures so successfully," Geoff said.

According to Geoff, a patient in the infusion center told him that he'd lose his desire for his favorite foods—burgers, Italian food and coffee. "While some things tasted funny, I still ate my burgers and fries," he said. He also continued taking his son to school and working, despite experiencing some nausea.

He added that, while he maintained his appetite, he lost his hair and his strength. He initially went to his local school to walk the track, and then he started to run. "Then I made it to a mile and walked and then ran some more. As long as I wasn't falling down, I pushed myself to getting back in shape," he remembers. One day his sister-in-law asked Geoff to enter a local 10K race called "The Great Cow Harbor Run," which he completed in a little over an hour wearing a t-shirt that graphically thanked his doctor.

His hair loss was a little more difficult to adjust to, especially for Geoff's son, who was nine at the time. "I explained the situation to him, and he'd ask me questions when he got curious," Geoff recalls. "One time he asked me if I'd wear a hat when I picked him up at school so I wouldn't scare his friends."

As if he wasn't undergoing enough change, Geoff also decided to change careers during this period. He left his position as an industrial chemicals salesperson, and underwent training to become a financial advisor.

During his stem cell replacement, he carted his laptop to the hospital and hooked it up to the telephone in the room to track the stock market on CNBC, monitor his accounts and keep in touch with his clients. "I didn't miss a beat," he said.

He does, however, still find time to relax by running, rollerblading, and playing golf and basketball. Geoff has also joined a buddy program through the American Cancer Society called 'Cansurmount,' in which he paired with newly diagnosed individuals with the same diagnosis to provide counseling and support.

"A lot of people really don't understand what they're going through and may be afraid to ask their doctor certain questions," Geoff explains. "I thought it was important for people to be able to talk to someone who was going through the same experience, so I attended the training class and have been a 'Cansurmount' patient volunteer ever since."

In his own experience and as a volunteer, he has come to appreciate the value of visualization in helping to overcome negative thoughts. "You can't keep wondering why you got this dread disease or questioning if God is punishing you," he advises. "Don't keep looking for the reason or the cause—just commit yourself to fight it with everything you have because you want to live."

Geoff suggests becoming more in tune with your body by controlling your breathing and your heart rate through exercise and yoga, and employing visualization exercises to imagine yourself ridding your body of cancer.

Some of the more effective ones he's encountered include exercises to visualize yourself forcing the cancer out of your body, seeing cancer as a gnarled black tree stump that is slowly uprooted and thrown away, and imagining yourself as a Star Wars fighter pilot shooting cancer cells with a laser.

In his own life, what Geoff visualizes is more worldly these days. "I'm glad to still be alive and to see my son growing up," he reports. "As for the other things, I'm confident they will all come in time."

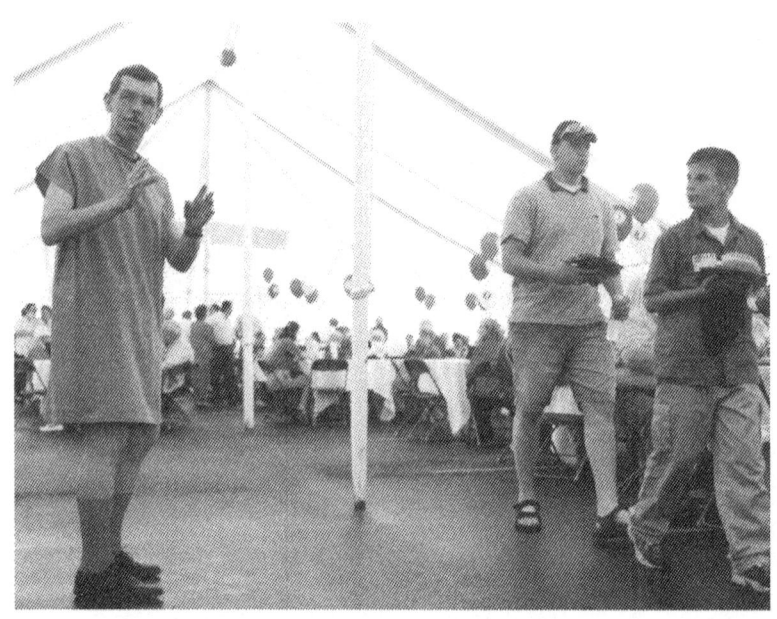

Larry Moore, 54

Married 32 years, with a daughter (24).

Larry is a supervisory auditor for the Department of Defense. He has both a CPA and an MBA.

Born: Fort Worth, TX. Lives: Arlington, TX.

Tumor Type: Myxoid liposarcoma (testicular), diagnosed 1978.

Treatment: Surgery to remove the right testicle and radiation.

Larry was the principal author of the handbook, "TEAMWORK: The Cancer Patient's Guide to Talking with Your Doctor" which is available through 888-650-9127 from the National Coalition for Cancer Survivorship in Silver Spring, Maryland. Over 300,000 copies have been distributed to cancer centers, hospitals, cancer patients, and support organizations. Larry can be reached for speaking engagements by email at larry@larrymoore.org

Photo Credit: Karen Vibert-Kennedy. Giving speech in 'patient garb'.

PERSISTENCE IN FINDING THE TRUTH

Ask questions and keep your chin up.

That's the advice of Larry Moore, a testicular cancer survivor whose illness had been misdiagnosed for five years.

"One doctor told me not to drive to the MD Anderson Cancer Center because it was 300 miles away," Larry recounts. "He was concerned about the inconvenience and hotel costs." He went anyway and was properly diagnosed.

As he entered surgery and radiation, "I thought I was going to die, but wanted to live more than anything because I had a wife and two-year-old daughter at the time," Larry remarked.

Six months after successful treatment, Larry ran his first marathon. "The longest I had ever run before my diagnosis was 10 miles," Mike said. "The White Rock Lake Marathon in Dallas was 26 miles. That was a really big deal for me." He has run seven more marathons since.

Larry stressed that individuals with cancer shouldn't be intimidated by their health care team. "Listen as carefully as you can and take notes," he advises, "and don't be afraid to break the medical language barrier." Larry also urges newly diagnosed patients not to be afraid of asking for copies of lab and surgical reports.

He continued, "Even if you're tactful, some doctors might take offense in your approach, but they'll get over it. But if you're not proactive and don't get the right information, *you* might not get over it," Larry warns. He insists that his own cancer treatment experiences saw both good and bad, but in either case demonstrated the critical importance of the doctor/patient relationship.

He also encourages optimism. "I've talked with hundreds of patients around the country and have heard countless stories of people who had incredible odds against them who've made it," he reflected.

Larry also stressed that fearing illness once you're through the initial cancer experience is all too common. "Every ache and pain scared me—you're always waiting for the other shoe to drop. But after you experience repeated scares and nothing happens—like X-rays that turn out to be false alarms—you become a bit more brave."

And sometimes, you just have to laugh. "Cancer is such a serious illness that you have to have a good sense of humor to survive," Larry said. In his public speaking engagements, he enters the stage in a hospital gown instead of traditional business attire. "When I come in a blue hospital gown, red socks and black shoes, I tell the audience that the program chairperson was looking for someone who could add a little dignity to the program," he says. "I then tell them that I figure I could add as little as anybody."

His rationale? "Cancer patients don't face cancer in a coat and tie, nor in an evening gown. Most of the time, they face it in a hospital gown, so that's how I speak to people to get their attention."

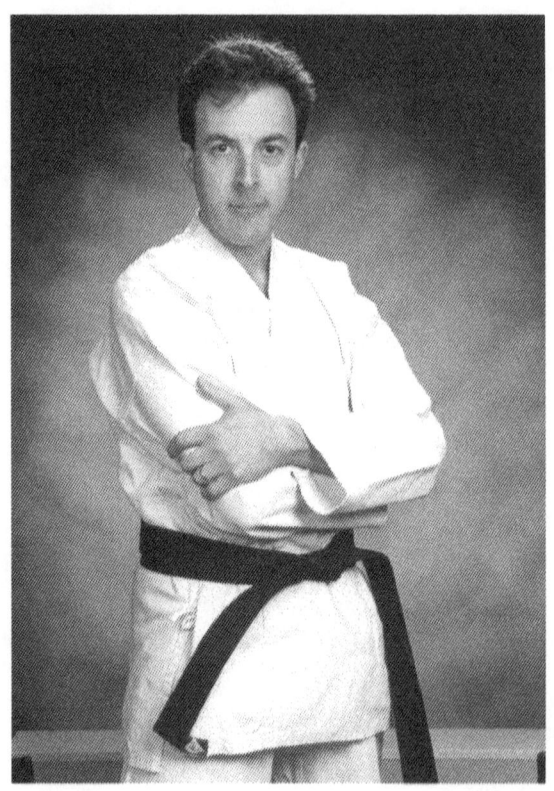

Barry Summers, 36

Married 6 years to Lorri, daughter Rachael (2).
Oncology Pharmaceutical Sales Representative for Ortho Biotech, a division of Johnson & Johnson.
Born: Philadelphia, PA; Live: Newtown, PA.
Tumor Type: stage two renal cell (kidney) carcinoma, diagnosed March 1997.
Treatment: Surgical removal of right kidney and adrenal gland.
Photo Credit: Unknown.

YOU SHOULD SEE THE OTHER GUY

A friendly jab in the ribs from a coworker may have saved Barry Summers' life.

"Her soft poke in the ribs actually broke my undiagnosed tumor, which caused my urine to turn brown," Barry said. "Having no other symptoms, I went to the doctor thinking I was dehydrated—he yelled at me for not coming in sooner. My urine was full of blood."

Barry had to wait nearly two weeks after his initial tests to see a urologist. "During this time, I had every bad dream imaginable. No one would say 'cancer', but I had a gut feeling," Barry said.

Barry was on the way to mail his test results to his brother, a radiologist, when he decided to take a peek himself. "My right kidney was four times larger than my left—right away I knew it was cancer," Barry remembers.

After the urologist diagnosed renal cell carcinoma, Barry's brother was his second opinion, and the surgery was scheduled for six days later. Unfortunately, he wasn't able to tell his wife ahead of time, and she learned of his cancer that afternoon as the on-call nurse at the blood draw unit where Barry had been instructed to self-donate prior to his surgery.

When he was diagnosed, Barry had been preparing to test for his Black Belt in karate, a goal he planned to realize before his 32nd birthday. "I was angry that my surgery would make me miss the date," Barry recounts. "My wife had to remind me that waiting two more months may have been too late. I wasn't able to see the bigger picture at the time."

Upon hearing that he'd be away for a few months, his karate sensei told Barry to meditate every night on getting better, advice that Barry says helped him tremendously.

He had his right kidney and adrenal gland removed, and was back in karate a few months later. "Less than seven months after my surgery, I got my Black Belt," Barry reports. "It was the most important thing I ever earned in my life."

Barry remembers changing into his karate uniform, when a new student noticed his fourteen-inch scar. "He was a little shocked, and I could tell he thought I got the injury in class," Barry recounts. "I told him, "You think I look bad, you should see the other guy!"

With his major goals achieved—his cancer removed and his Black Belt attained—Barry's day-to-day life became somewhat anti-climatic. "I attacked the depression with counseling and activity," Barry said. He became a Master-Instructor in the respected Japanese Healing Art known as "Reiki," built a brick patio in his back yard, painted a mural on the inside of his garage door and began to row on the Delaware River. His greatest accomplishment during this time, however, was fathering "a perfect little girl."

"She and her mom are the two best things that have ever happened to me," Barry reports.

Barry now realizes that, while he is the same person he was before he had cancer, his approach to life has changed. Throughout his experience, he was inspired by a fellow kidney cancer survivor who shared two thoughts with him. The first was a quote from the French writer Albert Camus: "In the depths of winter I find within me an invincible summer." The second was his friend's own words of wisdom. She told him, "When I get scared, I pretend my fear is a tiny box I'm holding in my fingers. I look at all sides of it and see how small it really is, and then I put it away in my pocket."

The story of Lance Armstrong's victory over testicular cancer and the Tour de France cycling race completed Barry's recovery, and is what lead him to compile this book of amazing cancer survivors.

"Some days all I need is to go sit on my patio, look at the trees or this little white farmhouse out in the distance, and know that peace really does flow through me," Barry said. "Cancer has made me stop here and change some things. While I can't ever get my kidney back, I can change how I do everything else moving forward."

0-595-20904-1